Register Now for Online Access to Your Book!

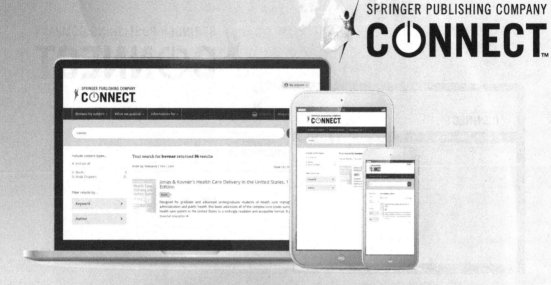

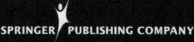

Register Now for Online Access to Your Book!

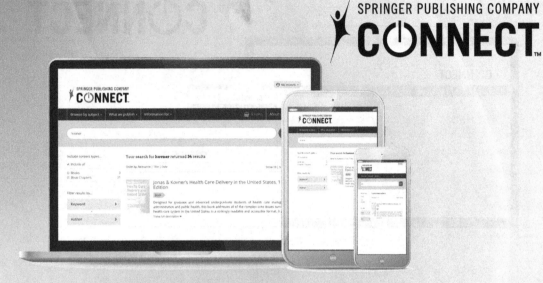

Your print purchase of *Case Studies in Global Health Policy Nursing*, **includes online access to the contents of your book**—increasing accessibility, portability, and searchability!

Access today at:
http://connect.springerpub.com/ content/book/978-0-8261-7211-2 or scan the QR code at the right with your smartphone and enter the access code below.

11FTHNWSD

Scan here for quick access.

Genie E. Dorman, PhD, RN, is a professor of nursing at Kennesaw State University WellStar School of Nursing. She has codirected study abroad programs in Mexico, Haiti, Puerto Rico, and the United Arab Emirates designed to enhance students' cultural competence through experiential learning. Her research interests include the provision of healthcare to the underserved and the development of cultural competence in both undergraduate and graduate students. She has made numerous presentations on these topics at both national and international conferences.

Mary de Chesnay, PhD, RN, PMHCNS-BC, FAAN, is a professor of nursing at Kennesaw State University, Kennesaw, Georgia. She is a former dean at Duquesne University and the first holder of the Jean Bushman Endowed Chair at Seattle University. She has extensive clinical experience in human trafficking, has taught health policy and research to graduate students, and has edited 10 books, 3 of which received the AJN Book of the Year award. She is the editor of the Springer Publishing series on qualitative research.

Case Studies in Global Health Policy Nursing

Genie E. Dorman, PhD, RN
Mary de Chesnay, PhD, RN, PMHCNS-BC, FAAN

Editors

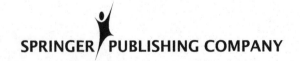

SPRINGER PUBLISHING COMPANY

Springer Publishing Company, LLC
11 West 42nd Street
New York, NY 10036
www.springerpub.com

Acquisitions Editor: Joseph Morita
Associate Managing Editor: Kris Parrish
Compositor: S4Carlisle Publishing Services

ISBN: 978-0-8261-7119-1
ebook ISBN: 978-0-8261-7211-2
Instructor's Resource Guide ISBN: 978-0-8261-7281-5
Instructor's PowerPoints ISBN: 978-0-8261-7311-9

Instructor's Materials: Qualified instructors may request supplements by emailing textbook@ springerpub.com.

18 19 20 21 22/5 4 3 2 1

The author and the publisher of this Work have made every effort to use sources believed to be reliable to provide information that is accurate and compatible with the standards generally accepted at the time of publication. The author and publisher shall not be liable for any special, consequential, or exemplary damages resulting, in whole or in part, from the readers' use of, or reliance on, the information contained in this book. The publisher has no responsibility for the persistence or accuracy of URLs for external or third-party Internet websites referred to in this publication and does not guarantee that any content on such websites is, or will remain, accurate or appropriate.

Library of Congress Cataloging-in-Publication Data

Names: Dorman, Genie, editor. | De Chesnay, Mary, editor.
Title: Case studies in global health policy nursing / Genie Dorman, Mary de
  Chesnay, editors.
Description: New York : Springer Publishing Company, [2018] | Includes
  bibliographical references and index.
Identifiers: LCCN 2018016744| ISBN 9780826171191 | ISBN 9780826172815
  (instructor's resource guide) | ISBN 9780826172112 (ebook) | ISBN 9780826173119
  (instructor's PowerPoints)
Subjects: | MESH: Health Policy | Global Health | Nurse's Role
Classification: LCC RT89 | NLM WA 530.1 | DDC 362.17/3--dc23 LC record available at
https://lccn.loc.gov/2018016744

Contact us to receive discount rates on bulk purchases.
We can also customize our books to meet your needs.
For more information please contact: sales@springerpub.com

Printed in the United States of America.

For Phillip and Kyle, and your unending patience and support.

GD

For Cynthia Elery, long-time administrative assistant to the Director of the School of Nursing, who keeps everything running smoothly.

MdC

Contents

Contributors

Jennifer Azelton, MSN, APRN, FNP-BC, completed her undergraduate nursing education at Chamberlain College of Nursing, receiving a BSN in 2010. She subsequently completed the WellStar Primary Care Nurse Practitioner Program at Kennesaw State University, receiving her MSN in 2016. She is currently employed as a certified family nurse practitioner.

Brenda Brown, DNS, RN, CNE, is a clinical instructor of nursing and a doctoral student at Kennesaw State University. Her doctoral focus is on the healthcare of women Afghan refugees. She has served as the Sigma Theta Tau International (STTI) ambassador to Afghanistan, and she is a volunteer with Georgia Refugee Health and Mental Health (GRHMH), an organization that provides healthcare to refugees.

Sharon Brownie, RN, RM, BEd, MEd Admin, M Hth S Mgt, MA Mgt (N), GAICD, FCNA, DBA, is the dean of nursing and midwifery at Aga Khan University, East Africa, where she provides leadership to campuses and faculty teams in Kenya and Tanzania. She has extensive management and leadership experience across the health, higher education, social, and business development sectors. Her executive leadership roles have included significant capacity building, workforce development, business growth, and change management mandates.

Adriana Caldwell, is a second-year biology student at Kennesaw State University. She has plans to go on to medical school to become a doctor in clinical pathology.

Jennifer Cooper, PhD, MSN, Post Grad Community Health, BSN, RN, has recently completed her doctorate in public health at Curtin University, Perth, Western Australia. She is a former nursing education/research manager/clinical resource nurse at Sheikh Khalifa Medical City, Abu Dhabi, United Arab Emirates. Her research interests include global health, in particular noncommunicable disease trends, program development, and management for the prevention of noncommunicable diseases.

Mary de Chesnay, PhD, RN, PMHCNS-BC, FAAN, is a professor of nursing at Kennesaw State University, Kennesaw, Georgia. She is a former dean at Duquesne University and the first holder of the Jean Bushman Endowed Chair at Seattle University. She has extensive clinical experience in human trafficking, has taught health policy and research to graduate students, and has edited 10 books, 3 of which received the AJN Book of the Year award. She is the editor of the Springer series on qualitative research.

Genie E. Dorman, PhD, RN, is a professor of nursing at Kennesaw State University WellStar School of Nursing. She has codirected study abroad programs in Mexico, Haiti, Puerto Rico, and the United Arab Emirates, designed to enhance students' cultural competence through experiential learning. Her research interests include the provision of healthcare to the underserved and the development of cultural competence in both undergraduate and graduate students. She has made numerous presentations on these topics at both national and international conferences.

Mari-Amanda Dyal, PhD, holds a doctorate in health promotion and behavior from the University of Georgia. Her research interests are rooted in workplace health promotion in the areas of job demands and job resources. Her health education and promotion background spans many specialties, settings, and populations. She is currently an assistant professor at Kennesaw State University for the Public Health Education program.

Jessica Ellis, RN, MSN, CNM, is a clinical assistant professor in the WellStar School of Nursing at Kennesaw State University and a PhD student in nursing at Georgia State University. Her research interests include reproductive health focusing on contraception and induction of labor.

Christie Emerson, DNSc, RN, is a clinical assistant professor in the WellStar School of Nursing at Kennesaw State University where she is also completing a doctorate in nursing science. In 2015, she was recognized by the Sultan Qaboos Cultural Center for her work toward the promotion of ties between the Sultanate of Oman and the United States of America. Her current research focuses on nurse leader perceptions of appropriate nurse staffing in Oman.

Janice Flynn, PhD, RN, is a professor of nursing at the WellStar School of Nursing at Kennesaw State University. She is a seasoned educator, with most of her teaching in adult health nursing. Her research has focused on online teaching and the genetics of breast cancer.

Elizabeth Holguin, MPH, MSN, FNP-BC, is a doctoral student at the University of New Mexico in nursing and health policy. She is a Robert Wood Johnson Foundation Nursing and Health Policy fellow and a Jonas Nurse Leader scholar. She served in the Peace Corps in Ethiopia and also implemented an infection control program in a government hospital in Kenema, Sierra Leone, West Africa.

Lorna Kendrick, PhD, APRN, PMHCNS-BC, is a UCLA graduate and is currently a tenured full professor and director of nursing at California State University San Marcos. She serves as archival secretary for the Council on Nursing and Anthropology (CONAA) of the Society for Applied Anthropology (SFAA). She has conducted ethnographic fieldwork and participatory action research with young African American men on untreated depression as a primary risk factor for early onset cardiovascular disease. Her research has taken her to destinations in Europe, Cuba, Alaska, Turkey, Argentina, Nigeria, and South Africa.

Jennifer M. Kilty, PhD, is associate professor in the Department of Criminology, University of Ottawa. Author of numerous journal articles and book chapters, she published *The Enigma of a Violent Woman: A Critical Examination of the Case of Karla Homolka* (Routledge) in 2016, and in 2014 she edited *Demarginalizing Voices: Commitment, Emotion and Action in Qualitative Research* (UBC Press) and *Within the Confines: Women and the Law in Canada* (Women's Press). From 2016 to 2017, she served as a Fulbright Visiting Research Chair at Kennesaw State University, conducting research on the criminalization of HIV nondisclosure.

R. Kevin Mallinson, PhD, RN, AACRN, FAAN,   is an associate professor and assistant dean for the doctoral division at the George Mason University School of Nursing in Fairfax, Virginia. He was the principal investigator for the Nurses SOAR! (Strengthening Our AIDS Response) nursing capacity–building program in southern Africa. He has more than 34 years of experience caring for persons with—or at risk for—HIV infection. He served as a Fulbright Scholar in the Kingdom of Swaziland for the 2012 to 2013 academic year, teaching and conducting research.

Krisola Marcano, MSN, APRN, FNP-BC,   is a foreign-trained physician who holds a doctor of medicine degree from the Universidad del Zulia in Venezuela. She has also completed both the undergraduate and graduate degree nursing programs at Kennesaw State University and is currently working as a family nurse practitioner in a private family practice. Her research interests include Latino decision making regarding immunizations.

Nancy Martinez, MSN, APRN, FNP-BC,   completed the WellStar School of Nursing BSN program in 2011. She subsequently completed the WellStar Primary Care Nurse Practitioner Program, receiving an MSN in 2016. She is currently working as a certified family nurse practitioner.

Jeri A. Milstead, PhD, RN, NEA-BC, FAAN,   is former dean and professor emerita, University of Toledo College of Nursing. She has worked in the public policy arena as advisor to a U.S. senator, taught policy to doctoral and master's students, and serves actively on boards, task forces, and committees in the public and private sectors. She has conducted research and consultation in the Netherlands, China, Jordan, Nicaragua, and Cuba. She is the editor and senior author of *Health Policy and Politics: A Nurse's Guide.*

Charlotte Ndema, MSN, APRN, FNP-BC,   holds a doctor of medicine degree from the University of Yaoundé, Cameroon, and a master of public health from Morgan State University. She completed both the undergraduate and graduate degree nursing programs at Kennesaw State University and currently works as a family nurse practitioner in Maryland.

Amy P. Roach, MSN, RN,   is a clinical assistant professor at Kennesaw State University WellStar School of Nursing. She is currently working on her dissertation to obtain her doctorate in nursing science. Her areas of research include transgender healthcare, health disparities, and access to healthcare for transgender individuals.

Donna Sabella, PhD, MEd, MSN, PMHNP-BC, is the Seedworks-endowed associate professor of social justice at the University of Massachusetts–Amherst College of Nursing and the cofounder and associate editor of the *Journal of Human Trafficking.* A former coordinator and creator of the Human Trafficking Certificate at Drexel University's College of Nursing and Health Professions, she is also a psychiatric nurse practitioner with experience working in corrections and with human trafficking victims.

Bongani T. Sibandze, MCur, RN, is a PhD student in the George Mason University School of Nursing in Fairfax, Virginia. Previously, he was a senior lecturer and Head of Department for Nursing, Faculty of Health Sciences at the Southern Africa Nazarene University in Manzini, Swaziland. Although he has experience conducting qualitative research, his dissertation research uses a mixed-methods design to explore the impact of professional nursing values on the caring behaviors of bedside nurses in Swazi hospitals.

M'Lyn Spinks, MSN, RN, is a part-time instructor of nursing in the WellStar School of Nursing at Kennesaw State University, where she is also currently pursuing a doctorate in nursing science. She received her MSN with a focus on nursing education from the University of West Georgia.

Johnathan D. Steppe, MSN, RN, is a clinical assistant professor in the WellStar School of Nursing at Kennesaw State University, where he is also pursuing a doctorate in nursing science. His clinical background is primarily in critical care. His current program of research focuses on health disparities in rural Nicaragua.

Evelina W. Sterling, PhD, is an assistant professor of sociology at Kennesaw State University. She earned a PhD in sociology from Georgia State University and a master's degree in public health from the Johns Hopkins University. She has 25 years of public health research experience focusing primarily on vulnerable populations and social factors in health.

Portia D. Thomas, MSN-CNE, MPH, is an epidemiologist for the Alabama Department of Public Health and also serves as an adjunct instructor at Virginia College in Montgomery, Alabama. Her nursing clinical specialty is medical surgical and research. Currently, she is a nursing doctoral student at Kennesaw State University where her program of research focuses on HIV prevention in men who have sex with men.

Foreword

We find ourselves in a world where healthcare is now a political platform, where gaps in healthcare services exist worldwide for a vast number of reasons. We find ourselves at a point in our professional history where hospitals should no longer be the primary locations to train our nurses or other healthcare professionals for the future. The current trend is moving toward hospitals requiring pay per each student they allow into their facility.

As a society, we find ourselves living on the next rung of a microwave paradigm where we want what we want now. It is no longer avant-garde to patiently go through the process of becoming a well-rounded liberal arts–trained future employee by learning the skills you need for the next 10 to 20 years out in your profession of choice. This growth process, known as a liberal arts education, is where one learns to be a stellar decision maker through the lessons learned in history and a person of integrity through the lessons learned debating ethical and moral issues.

Many of today's students are choosing programs not associated with liberal arts universities. Instead, their goals are to finish fast, get on with their careers, and increase their earning potential. In addition, the liberal arts schools find themselves competing with the nontraditional programs as well. The liberal arts programs are feeling forced to decrease the length of their programs. With decreased program length, many valuable courses and experiences are eliminated. The content within these courses was designed specifically to facilitate personal and professional transformation by instilling an attitude of lifelong learning, inclusivity, and respect for the lives, beliefs, and choices of others.

Initially, a global focus among nursing programs was often found in nursing programs with a faith-based history. The goals were to broaden students' worldviews and teach them the value of being others centered through missions and service. Many faculty from these faith-based schools and faculty born outside our county and wanting to give back to their country of origin shared their passion for global health with colleagues. This shared passion among colleagues turned into the global initiatives we see across the nation in most universities today.

An additional advantage of the global focus on practice has fostered policy changes led by nurses who, before their global experiences, were satisfied caring for patients in hospitals. Now, having experienced alternative practices, ideology, and environments, those nurses found themselves advocating for change, for help, for funding, and for a wealth of concepts they hadn't had to focus on at the bedside. These global experiences helped nurses see the challenges of food/home insecurities, of the working poor, of working uninsured, as well as of the undocumented uninsured person needing care.

As a society and citizens of the world, we nurses can no longer retain a narrow view of health and healthcare. We can no longer continue to limit our training and education to a hospital-based focus. As healthcare professionals, we are challenged by new disease strains that cross continental divides. The training we provide our future care providers needs to change. Supplemental and updated trainings are also needed for those who have already completed their education. Currently, the training nursing students complete has not changed in over 50 years. It is time to view health and healthcare from a world or global lens. The chapters and content within this book, *Case Studies in Global Health Policy Nursing*, provide an opportunity to add to the lens with which we train our future care providers.

Through service and global learning experiences, students' worldviews are broadened in ways traditional education is left wanting. Students with experiences inclusive of boundless classroom walls become critical thinkers, stellar decision makers, and limitless leaders. These same students go on to become activists for change, and thus these change agents are the innovators behind the development of policies needed to alter the status quo within society.

The nursing profession, among others, focused on whole-person care became one of the greatest proponents for providing healthcare to the world. Nurses have historically answered the call to travel to other countries in response to a variety of world emergencies. These experiences caring for others within our local and world communities have opened the eyes of many nurses to the atrocities occurring in our own backyards as well as around the world. This awareness alters the lives of both the provider and the recipient of care.

Traditionally, global health has depended predominately on local guides as well as the past experiences of a cadre of people, from other medical personnel to researchers and anthropologists, to name a few. There are few books available that offer students or others traveling the world to care for those experiencing healthcare challenges. This book provides the valuable content needed in preparation for or in tandem with a global experience. Dorman and de Chesnay offer a wealth of valuable information students and other healthcare providers would normally not receive until they were in the trenches of their global experience.

Dorman and de Chesnay deliver an overview in *Case Studies in Global Health Policy Nursing* of information that care providers would need to understand related policies across continents, nuances of ideology about care and disease from various countries, and what global health policy entails and means to healthcare providers traveling the world, along with case studies from several guides/experienced global experts.

Within the traditions of nursing, there are still those who believe student experiences should be at the bedside within the confines of hospitals. These same traditionalists view courses such as community health or mental health care as specialty areas, which expose students to those areas to a degree, but are not the primary focus of nursing education. What many traditionalists overlook is the global experiences that can teach students the intricacies of bedside care and assessment as well as allow a seamless incorporation of mental health, discharge planning, critical thinking, patient teaching, and most importantly personal growth and maturity.

I commend my colleagues Drs. Dorman and de Chesnay for their trailblazing text and their willingness to deliver a book we can use as the guide to begin conversations in classrooms among our future care providers about the importance of global health policy at home and around the world.

Lorna Kendrick, PhD, APRN, PMHCNS-BC
Professor and Director, School of Nursing
California State University San Marcos

Preface

Global health policy should be of interest to nurses and other providers involved in all aspects of healthcare, including practice, education, and administration. The overall purpose of this book is to disseminate policy analysis of key health issues that have a global impact from the perspective of nurses. The book is a compilation of case studies that highlight global initiatives to eradicate disease and promote health. The contributors are nurses who possess expertise in the global implications of the health issues and related policies of selected topics. Some of the topics included are transgender health, immigrant healthcare, chronic disease, human trafficking, pandemics, and infection control. These topics, as well as the others covered, are timely and of global significance. The case study approach provides the reader with an in-depth treatment of each topic's health issue and the global policy implications.

There are many textbooks regarding global implications of health policy, but our goal here is to provide the unique perspective of nurses who live and work with these implications as they strive to provide care and educate future nursing professionals. Because the case studies presented provide an overview of a variety of significant global health issues and the policies that impact them, the book is appropriate for students of public health and medical anthropology/sociology as well as graduate nursing students.

Qualified instructors may obtain access to ancillary materials, including an instructor's resource guide and PowerPoint presentations, by emailing textbook@springerpub.com.

Genie E. Dorman
Mary de Chesnay

Acknowledgments

As in any publishing endeavor, there were numerous people involved in the creation of this final draft. The contributors shared their varied experiences as educators, administrators, and providers in global health policy presented as case studies. In their eclectic roles, each brought a unique perspective to the significant effects that policy issues have on global health.

In addition, we are greatly indebted to Joseph Morita and Rachel Landes, the great people at Springer Publishing Company who oversaw this project and supported and guided us throughout the process. We are also indebted to the people who proofed the work and created the hard copies, including Vinolia Benedict Fernando at S4Carlisle Publishing Services.

At Kennesaw State University, Dr. Tommie Nelms, the former director of the WellStar School of Nursing (WSON), was a never-ending source of support and encouragement. In addition, there were several members of the WSON administrative team whose efforts were essential in the completion of this work. These include Cynthia Elery, assistant to the director and office manager; Jennifer Dawkins, graduate student services coordinator; Lindsey McKenzie, administrative assistant; and Mollett McCloud, administrative assistant.

General Topics

Policy Implications for Global Health

Jeri A. Milstead

To think today that health issues in one country are confined to that country indicates a lack of understanding of disease transmission, cultural practices, and migration patterns at the least. McLuan and Fiore's (1968) observation that it takes a village to raise a child certainly can be extrapolated to today's observation that a health problem in one country (or province or state) probably has an impact or corollary in at least one other country or area. In this chapter, the author presents health problem issues and policies that impact populations around the globe. To highlight the worldwide impact, the content is framed within the seven continents. The health issues are not exclusive but selected to reflect the extent of political or governmental impact.

Government structures are described briefly, and an overview of the policy-making process of the country examined is presented. The policy process will vary among countries depending on the type of government. We ask how the citizen voice is heard. Some issues may reflect cultural practices that may not be amenable to government intervention. The reader should determine the extent to which citizens, especially nurses, can be involved in the policy process as advocates and change agents.

AFRICA

Geographically, Africa can be divided into sub-Saharan regions (countries south of the Sahara Desert) and North Africa (countries north of the Sahara Desert and considered part of the League of Arab States). Sub-Sahara Africa includes countries on the western hump of the continent (Mauritania, Somalia, Djibouti, and Comoros that are considered part of the League of Arab States but are not situated in North Africa). Governments on this continent range from democracy to dictatorship to anarchy.

Nigeria, a tropical country, is situated on the west coast of Africa and borders on the Gulf of Guinea. Home to approximately 150 million people, Nigeria has the largest population of any country or territory on the continent. Following the transition from British colonial rule and several strong military takeovers, the current government is a presidential democracy with executive, legislative, and judicial components. The legislative branch, known as the National Assembly, comprises a House of Representatives (Green Chamber) of 251 members and a Senate (Red Chamber) of 109 members (Brown, 2013; Constitution of Nigeria, 1999). The government is "characterized by ethno-religious politics" (Brown, 2013, p. 173); that means that decisions made by bureaucratic leaders and political parties reflect cultural, often tribal, values that may not benefit necessarily a broad population.

The greatest health problem on this continent is the continuing growth of HIV/AIDS. Sub-Saharan Africa has nearly 70% of the world's HIV/AIDS population; Nigeria has 3.5 million people living with HIV; approximately 160,000 Nigerians died from AIDS in 2016 (avert.org/professionals/hiv-around-world/sub-saharan-africa/nigeria). The Nigerian federal government developed a 5-year National Strategic Plan (NSP) on HIV and AIDS in 2010, and the president initiated a Presidential Comprehensive Response Plan (PCRP) in 2013 with a target of preventing 105,000 new HIV infections. To date, an account of goal achievement has not been reported (www.avert.org).

Men who have sex with men (MSM) are much more at risk of HIV than the general population (Vu et al., 2013). MSM are the fastest growing group for new HIV infections though there are stringent laws against homosexuality. Punishment of up to 14 years in prison is not the only law; anyone who assists a homosexual person or couple faces up to 10 years in prison. For this reason, many men do not get tested, so never seek treatment. People who inject drugs (PWID) account for nearly 10% of new HIV infections. PWID are mostly women and are "seven times more likely to be living with HIV than their male counterparts"

(p. 3). Harm reduction services, such as needle/syringe exchanges and drug substitution are not available in Nigeria. Condom distribution and education about transmission of HIV and hepatitis C are provided but, because of the stigma of HIV/AIDS, are not used often.

Barriers that prevent testing, transmission, and treatment of HIV/AIDS include:

- Legal—The fear of imprisonment for homosexual activity is a very real barrier to testing.

- Social/cultural—Human rights for women are discriminatory. For example, females have some land rights but only males can inherit and own land. Women are under pressure to give birth to boys who can own land, which leads to having many children and not using contraceptives. This increases a woman's risk for contracting HIV (Avert, 2017, p. 6).

- Structural—Not only are there few or no government services available but universal precautions are not required and policies related to the safety of blood and blood products are inadequate.

- Economic—The Nigerian Agency for the Control of AIDS (NACA) surveys the population but does not provide services. Most funding for health programs in Nigeria comes from international sources. For example, the Global Fund to Fight AIDS, Malaria and Tuberculosis provided funding for all three programs, but suspended financial support after an audit of NACA uncovered millions of dollars in fraud and collusion (Avert, 2017, p. 6).

Africa's early response to the HIV/AIDS healthcare crisis was profound silence that was illustrated by persons not getting tested or treated, communities not discussing the disease and stigmatizing those they thought had the disease, and officials not mobilizing resources to address the problem (Population Reference Bureau, 2002). In 2002, wives of 18 African presidents met with United Nations officials in Switzerland to discuss what the women could do to persuade the governments to put more resources into the crisis.

With the exception of South Africa's president, Thabo Mbeki, who did not believe that HIV caused AIDS ("Mibeki Digs in," 2000) and who initiated government policies that banned retroviral medications to HIV-positive citizens, most sub-Sahara African countries eventually developed strategies to reduce the stigma surrounding those with HIV/AIDS.

Religious leaders in the 1990s favored only abstinence outside marriage and fidelity inside marriage, discrimination that exerted great influence, especially in the rural communities (Ucheaga & Hartwig, 2010). By 2010, the Nigerian government had worked with faith-based groups, international organizations, LGBTI alliances, and the media to create the National HIV/AIDS Stigma Reduction Strategy, and the latest survey reports that discrimination is becoming less each year (National HIV/AIDS Stigma Reduction Strategy, 2017).

Although HIV/AIDS is the most pressing disease at this time, one must not forget the Ebola and polio outbreaks. The first case of Ebola occurred in Lagos, Nigeria—the largest city in Africa. Described as a "powder keg" because of its crowded, poor population, many of whom live in slums, Lagos was a perfect setting for a devastating, apocalyptical crisis. Nigerian governmental officials, the U.S. Centers for Disease Control and Prevention (CDC), the World Health Organization (WHO), and many others provided huge amounts of resources (money, mobile phones, healthcare professionals, isolation quarters) to the city and other parts of the country. Despite hundreds dying, the situation was contained ("Nigeria now is free of Ebola," 2014). On the other hand, recent outbreaks of polio have been reported. No cases of wild poliovirus type 1 (WPV1) have been reported in 2017, but a new strain called circulating vaccine-derived poliovirus type 2 (cVDPV2) has prompted a concerted effort to vaccinate children, especially those in the more rural areas where access to healthcare is sparse (Polio Global Eradication Initiative, 2018).

LEARNING ACTIVITIES

1. What current policies (governmental and non-governmental) can assist the prevention of HIV/AIDS?

2. What governmental policies and resources could improve access so that the population is tested and treated?

3. What would it take to change the laws in Nigeria related to homosexuality?

4. What is needed to strengthen economic policies to sustain programs?

5. What stakeholders are needed to assist women to change the culture, so that women will have a stronger voice in their personal lives and become involved in setting policy?

6. What telemedicine technologies could bring services to remote areas of the country?

7. What evidence would indicate a strong commitment in resources and collaboration among the private sector and federal, state, and local governmental funding?

ANTARCTICA

The continent of Antarctica is an anomaly—there are no indigenous people and no government "No nation owns Antarctica" (United States Antarctic Program, 2016–2018, p. 1). There are many people from countries around the globe who work in science laboratories on a short-term basis for less than a year (www.dri.edu). Fifty-two countries have signed the Antarctica Treaty that requires agreement with basic health-related practices. Scientists, journalists, and educators live within the health policies of their own disparate countries; some countries require vaccinations of various types, others do not. "There are no natural severe diseases in Antarctica" (p. 8). People bring with them risks of many diseases, so most countries (or at least businesses and academic institutions) require a basic set of immunizations before coming to the continent.

People who work in Antarctica live in close quarters, often on ships or in confined spaces, that increase the risk of exposure to many diseases. Some ships have a physician or dentist on board. People who share facilities (showers, bathrooms, eating utensils) are likely to come down with common diseases and pass them on quickly. Unless isolated quickly, a disease can be transmitted to others quickly.

Academic institutions often interview researchers and educators prior to approving an assignment to Antarctica to be sure that the personnel are aware and have the capacity to cope with long winters, little sunshine, close quarters, and little variation in living conditions. According to a British Antarctica Survey Medical Unit (BASMU), conditions that usually preclude assignment to the continent include diabetes, lower limb amputation, malaria, hepatitis B, and HIV/AIDS, and any psychiatric diagnosis. Most health-related problems come from frostbite and hypothermia caused by subfreezing temperatures and winds (www.dri.edu), broken bones and sprains from falling on ice, and snow blindness (United States Antarctic Program, 2016–2018, pp. 55–58). Polar stations contain first-aid manuals that address carbon dioxide poisoning from cerebral edema that may occur at high altitudes (United States Antarctic Program, n.d.).

Since there is no official government, cooperation among countries and personnel is essential. The Antarctic Treaty, created in 1959 by 12 nations to ensure peaceful international research, has become a nongovernmental regulatory system that now includes environmental protection components (U.S. Department of State, n.d.). Recognition of common health-related problems is necessary. Acknowledgment of policies from many countries that address the prevention, diagnosis, and treatment of potential or actual problems requires trust and respect. The unique mandatory cooperative characteristic of this continent highlights the need for planning before assignment and cooperation at the site. If a worker develops a health problem that needs to be treated at the home country, on-site personnel may have to handle the situation until transportation can be arranged, which can be months. Frequent bad weather conditions (blizzards, subfreezing temperatures, high winds) may not allow planes to fly or ships to sail.

LEARNING ACTIVITIES

1. Identify health-related policies relevant to Antarctica from your own country, academic institution, or business. Consider how you would implement these policies before and after you land on this continent.

2. How could current technology be used to address health problems on this continent?

3. What types of healthcare professionals would be most valuable on a research or educational expedition to this continent? Why?

4. How would you treat a person who develops an acute health problem?

5. What special training would you expect before signing on to a trip to this continent?

6. How would you go about developing a policy related to maintaining good health on Antarctica? What resources would you need to develop this policy?

ASIA

This section of the chapter will explore India, the second largest country in Asia (China being the largest), because of the density of the population and the burden on the healthcare system. India is projected to surpass China in population by 2022 (United Nations, 2015, p. 4). This large country is a sovereign, socialist, democratic republic. After occupation by the Portuguese, Dutch, French, and a long rule by the British, India gained independence in 1947. The population is approximately 1.3 billion, with 41% between the ages of 25 and 54 (World Factbook, 2017). Eighty percent are Hindus, and Hindi is the language spoken mostly, although English is used for governmental, political, and business purposes (Central Intelligence Agency, 2018).

The government consists of three branches: executive (president, vice-president, and the cabinet), parliamentary legislative system, and a judiciary (supreme court and lesser state courts; www.elections.in/government). A constitution adopted in 1950 espoused a right to life for all citizens but fell short of guaranteeing a right to health. There are 545 members of the Lok Sabha (lower house) and 250 members of the Rajya Sabha (upper house) of Parliament. The representation of women in either house is only 11%, far below the average of 193 parliaments in the world (Sengupta, 2017). Women's rights traditionally have not been strong. Women have not had access to higher education, in part due to the caste system.

India historically has had a clear system of social stratification that is tied to Hinduism. Brahmins (from God Brahma's head) are the elite and were accepted as scholars and religious leaders. They were eligible for college and were considered superior to other humans. The next level in the hierarchy are rulers and warriors (from Brahma's arms, a reflection of Indian history of oppression and dependence), then merchants, farmers, and those in the trades (from the god's thighs). Following that are the lowest level of laborers (from the God's feet), such as street sweepers and latrine cleaners, often known as the untouchables. A separate classification named Scheduled Tribes are those people who have refused to live in cities and towns and who still live in the jungles and mountains (BBC, 2016; Taseer, 2016). One is born into a caste and, until the mid-20th century, could never move upward. In 1950, during the break from British rule that coincided with civil rights movements in many countries, discrimination based on caste and other designations was declared illegal. However, the caste system still exists unofficially because this system is so deeply rooted in the culture; there remains a subtle and not-so-subtle reality noted in stereotypes.

The health system in India is structured and administered by government. States carry the burden of providing care but funding is inconsistent, and there are not enough educated and trained providers. A "triple burden" of communicable, non-communicable, and emerging infectious diseases places a load on government resources (Chauhan, 2011, p. 89). India spends only 1% of its gross domestic product (GDP) on health, far less than most developed countries. Technically, preventive primary care, diagnostic services, and in- and out-patient hospital care is free, but realistically there are not enough trained and educated providers, and access to care and medication is severely restricted. Seventy percent of health expenditures are paid out of pocket by patients (Chauhan, 2011, p. 91; Mossialos & Wenzel, 2015). Even though India has the highest rate of tuberculosis in the world and endured an outbreak of the plague in 1994, the highest mortality rates come from non-communicable diseases. Cardiovascular problems, chronic obstructive pulmonary disease (COPD) and asthma, cancer, and senility are the most frequent health problems (Chauhan, 2011, p. 90).

In 2017, a National Health Policy was enacted that moves healthcare from a strictly public system to a public–private partnership. Prevention of disease and disability and health promotion are the cornerstones. The goal is to provide access to quality healthcare for all citizens (Gupta & Bhatia, 2017). Special focus will be on mental health (7% of the population has mental health needs) and testing, diagnosis, and treatment for HIV/AIDS. The future looks bright legally, but much of the success or failure for health programs will be due to the amount of sustained funding and the depth of education and training made available.

LEARNING ACTIVITIES

1. Given the democratic philosophy of India, how can more citizens get their health issues on the national agenda so that they can obtain a government response? List tactics to raise consciousness about issues. List ways to define a health issue for different stakeholders.

2. Identify at least two members of Parliament in each chamber who could be persuaded to introduce legislation to address

one major health problem. Construct a one-page fact sheet about your issue with information about a contact in case there are questions.

3. Role-play a visit to a member of Parliament in which you present your issue. State facts, a brief background of the health problem, how many of the member's constituents are affected, and a personal story. Expect the visit to last approximately 5 to 10 minutes.

4. Create a proposal for a baccalaureate and advanced nurse education program. What resources would you use? What colleagues could you include to assist you with accreditation issues and national standards? How would you explain the value of these professionals to the health system?

AUSTRALIA

Australia, a continent and developed country, is a constitutional monarchy with three distinct divisions of government: executive, legislative, and judiciary. The English monarch (i.e., Queen Elizabeth) is the titular head of state who appoints a governor-general (GC) to serve as head of government (executive branch). A parliamentary branch of elected representatives (ministers) from all states and eight territories and a judiciary complete the central structure that provides political checks and balances. The GC works with the prime minister, who is responsible for making policy. State and local governments are the functional units where policies are implemented (www.aph.gov.au, www.australia.gov.au/about). The governmental structure illustrates a democracy in which citizens can participate at the local, state, and federal levels.

Healthcare is provided by public and private services. The Australian government has a national health policy called Medicare that is government funded and guarantees healthcare services for all. Physician visits, medical care (blood tests, etc.), and pharmaceuticals are the responsibility of the federal level; hospital care is managed at the state level (www.australia.gov.au/information-and-services/health). Patients pay no fees or co-payments for care. Patients may choose a private care option but that is paid out of pocket.

Health priorities vary, depending on who is reporting. In 2014, three of the top medical experts in the country listed the top most important health issues from their specific perspective (www.ama.com.au/ausmed/five-most-pressing-health-priorities-2014). The governmental chief medical officer listed antimicrobial resistance, emerging infectious diseases, and immunization coverage as the three most important items on his list. The president of the Australian Medical Association recognized population health as a cross-portfolio (i.e., interprofessional) issue throughout all levels of government, investing in the gap between Aboriginal and Torre Strait Islanders and all Australians, and expansion of e-health. A third perspective on health priorities was issued by a visiting fellow from the Australian Primary Care Research Institute who believes that addressing health disparities, changing the payment method for healthcare services, and realigning the workforce are most important (Moore, 2016). This same year, the Australian Institute of Health and Welfare (AIHW) reported that the leading cause of ill health is chronic disease. Within that category are cardiovascular disease, cancer, COPD, and diabetes; diseases that represent 75% of disease-related deaths (https://www.aihw.gov.au/reports/life-expectancy-death/deaths-in-australia/contents/multiple-causes-of-death). Harrison, Henderson, Miller, and Britt (2017) reported the six chronic health issues that affected Australians are hypertension, hyperlipidemia, depression, diabetes, anxiety, and asthma and that 40% of Australians had at least one of the conditions.

The Australian healthcare system faces serious challenges (Macri, 2016). Funding is becoming a burden to citizens as taxes increase. Taxes fund health services, so physician visits and hospital care are strained. A growing aging population has long-term chronic conditions that require more services. Expensive technology has become essential to gathering and organizing data to improve the coordination of care among providers, structures, and populations. As noted above, a lack of alignment of health priorities has a fragmented effect on funding. The care available to indigenous people falls short of the general population, partly because of lack of access in remote areas such as central Australia.

Health expert Mark Britt believes that the current federal-state structure of providing services is old-fashioned and in need of updating. He also highlighted that payment for physicians must move from a fee-for-service system and that care must become better coordinated. This "triple whammy" of concerns must be addressed through the involvement of citizens who engage with their government representatives. Citizens must use the political arena to address serious health issues (Gardner, 2015).

LEARNING ACTIVITIES

1. Consider who speaks for underserved populations. How do advocates obtain correct data?

2. How can advocates separate their own biases from issues of diverse populations?

3. Identify stakeholders who could assist you with advocating for change in governmental policies and programs.

4. Argue persistence versus need for action now in setting and changing policy.

EUROPE

Europe is a huge landmass between the Arctic Circle (north), Mediterranean Sea (south), Atlantic Ocean (west), and Asia (east). The continent comprises 50 countries, 28 of which are members of the European Union, an alliance of countries since 1993. The European Council sets the policy agenda and priorities for the members. The governance structure consists of the Council of the EU (executive functions), the European Parliament (laws and regulations), and the European Judiciary (www.citizensinformation.ie/en). Member countries came together to present a more unitary position to the economic world. Many legal and regulatory changes have evolved, such as the relaxation of border control. Each country also has its own government.

ITALY

So far, this chapter has presented health problems in various countries. However, there are areas in the world where good health is enjoyed despite a lack of government resources or policies. Italy is the focal point for presentation of health issues in Europe. Instead of examining health challenges, we will look at a country that has been named the healthiest of 163 countries surveyed by Bloomberg (Lu & DelGiudice, 2017a) and the healthiest of 25 countries surveyed by CEO World Magazine (Dhirag, 2017). Italy is a constitutional democratic republic with three independent sections: executive (Council of Ministers, president), legislative (two-chamber Parliament), and a judiciary (over which the president presides). Citizens have the right to vote to directly elect the 630 deputies (lower chamber) and 315 senators (upper chamber). Bills may be introduced by members of Parliament and the president/Council of Ministers.

The economy is depressed—exports have decreased since 2010; infrastructure is old and deteriorating. For example, the lack of upgrading of the ports has led to a devastating decrease in international trade, and the railroads are so ancient that they are not reliable. The northern and southern regions exhibit very different levels of growth and prosperity. Between 2007 and 2014, 70% of employment was found in the south, although only 33% of workers in the region are women (50% nationally; Lu & DelGiudice, 2017b).

The healthcare system consists of universal coverage funded by employer-based taxes; no one may opt out. The system is directed by the 19 major regions of the country and is administered at the local level. Because of the great differences in industrialization between the northern and southern areas of the country, there are major discrepancies in the quality, accessibility, and cost of healthcare (Lu & DelGiudice, 2017b). Healthcare in the south is focused on sickness, not prevention and promotion of health (Donatini, 2016). Regular health check-ups are not available and services are not uniform.

So, why is the country that has such a poor economy and a poorly funded and operated healthcare system considered to be the healthiest in the world? The southern culture is one in which the stress level is not high (despite the poor job market). The diet is a Mediterranean style consisting of tomato-based sauces, fish (especially anchovies), extra virgin olive oil, and the use of rosemary and oregano. The activity level is slow (Santevecchi, 2016). The northern people enjoy a moderate climate with access to fresh vegetables and vineyards but face unemployment due to a depressed economy.

LEARNING ACTIVITIES

1. What research questions would you construct in proposing to study reasons for a healthy population in spite of economic challenges?

2. Even though the economy revolves around an outdated manufacturing system with lost jobs, why would not that system cause increased stress that might lead to poor health?

3. Discuss the impact of diet as a significant factor in good health.

4. Identify strategies that could improve the administration of health services at the regional and local levels. Research possible barriers such as education and work opportunities for men and women.

5. Develop an evaluation plan that addresses efficiency and effectiveness of the healthcare system.

NORTH AMERICA

North America is composed of two countries (Canada and the United States) and a third area of several countries (Central America). Weather ranges from arctic to tropical. Governments mostly are democracies but there is much diversity within each country/area. This segment reviews the common health problems of American Indians/Alaska Natives (AIAN). The term AIAN, used by the U.S. 2010 Census, refers to "a person having origins in any of the original peoples of North and South America (including Central America) and who maintains a tribal affiliation or community attachment" (United States Census, 2010). Other acceptable terms noted by AIAN include First People, Original People, and Indigenous People but do not include derogatory terms such as squaw, redskin, and savage (www.indiancountrymedianetwork.com). The approximately five million who declare themselves AIAN make up 2% of the U.S. population (Artigan, Arguello, & Duckett, 2013).

The leading causes of death in the United States in 2017 are cardiovascular disease, cancer, and accidents (www.cdc.gov/nchs/products/databriefs/db293.htm). Gone and Trimble (2012) report the significant healthcare needs of AIAN involve treatment for depression, diabetes, and cardiovascular disease (the latter identified as causing the most deaths; www.rwjf.org). Artigan et al. (2013) reported that one third are below the age of 19 years (26% in the U.S. population) and that only 7% are over the age of 65 years. Sarche and Spicer report that AIAN children have the "highest rate of violence and trauma involving serious injury to themselves or other whom they know" (2008, p. 128). Suicide is the second leading cause of death in adolescents and young adults.

All AIAN have access to healthcare through facilities administered through the non-urban Indian Health Service (IHS; Artiga, Arguello, & Duckett, 2013). A problem of health disparities exists because most IHS services are provided on reservations and 67% of AIAN live in U.S. cities, not on reservations where services are located; only 22% live on reservations or land trusts. Designated contract health services (CHS) may be available in some private non-urban hospitals but are limited to emergency care for life-threatening conditions. "Individuals who rely solely on IHS or are without any form of health insurance coverage are classified by the U.S. government as uninsured." Nearly 60% of IHS services go for direct care provided by tribes—only 1% of total program dollars are spent on urban health services.

IHS funding must be appropriated by the Congress every year—a process that seems set up to discourage continuing funding, let alone approval of any increases. Historically, IHS is underfunded. Medicaid fills the gap, but Medicaid is a federal-state matching program in which funds depend on each state's allocation. Therefore, AIAN are subjected to limited services based on how near they are or if they can obtain transportation to tribal facilities.

LEARNING ACTIVITIES

1. Create a one-page fact sheet to present to those in Congress and the Senate that highlights the serious nature of AIAN health issues and lack of IHS funding.

2. Identify stakeholders who can accompany AIAN leaders to policy makers' offices to discuss issues, request policy changes, and request funding.

3. What kinds of health professionals are needed in IHS facilities to address the most serious needs of AIAN?

4. Discuss with local AIANs their cultural beliefs and traditions related to health. For example, are there tribal curanderos or others who provide non-traditional care? Are they effective?

SOUTH AMERICA

Instead of selecting one country in South America, this segment will focus on the whole continent. There are 14 countries and 433.5 million people in a geographic area of 6.888 million miles (worldometers, 2017). There are three sub-regions: Andean, tropical, and southern (Mercer, 2015). Spanish is the language of most countries, although Portuguese is the language of Brazil. Government systems vary from democracy to dictatorship.

Literature on health issues focuses on children. All countries signed a declaration to protect human rights (Mercer, 2015). This agreement guaranteed the right to health for every child. In spite of this, the mortality rate for children from birth to 5 years is very high because of widespread poverty. A pervasive religious presence forbids birth control, and the incidence of pregnancy in young girls is high. Typically, a very young girl does not have a body mature enough to carry a fetus to term so often delivers prematurely. Low birth weight babies frequently require neonatal intensive care that may not be available or may be very expensive. However, the infant mortality rate (IMR) for the continent decreased by 67% between 1990 and 2015. During the same period, the maternal mortality rate (MMR) also decreased by 75%. The dramatic decreases are due to a more robust economy that allowed more government assistance programs to the poor (Health in South America, 2012). Argentina, Chile, and Uruguay had a high level of economic development at the time and provided a higher level of assistance than countries that were still struggling such as Bolivia, Paraguay, or Peru.

The reduction in mortality rates has altered the statistics on the causes of death and disease. Although there is a strong correlation between level of education and poverty, accidents, tobacco/alcohol/drug use, and unprotected sexual behavior remain the top three causes of injury and illness to children 10 to 19 years old. There is consensus that major problems are seen in chronic malnutrition and anemia, obesity, perinatal disorders, accidents, violence, and sexually transmitted diseases. There still is much child labor, street begging, sexual trafficking, and criminal gangs. Mercer sees in this continuing crisis some prospects for action. Most statistics provided are averages, which disguise the huge gap between the health of indigent and non-indigent people (Mercer, 2015).

One ray of hope comes in the form of a South American indigenous tribe that was discovered to have the "healthiest hearts ever studied" ("South American Tribe," 2017). A research group from the University of New Mexico, headed by Hillard Kaplan, studied the Tsimane who live in the Bolivian Amazon area and found that the natives had zero risk for heart disease. A diet of complex carbohydrates, wild game and fish, and little fat or protein and strenuous daily activity throughout the life span are reported to be the foundation for their remarkable condition.

Corruption and violence have been the norm in most South American countries. Political coups, anti-government protests, firebombed buildings, and sabotaged transportation systems are common occurrences (Miroff, 2017). During the 20th century, oil and iron ore were major exports. In the 21st century, competition from other countries/continents has driven down the price of these commodities with a resultant reduction in income and an increase in taxes in most South American countries. The population became increasingly distrustful of "big government" and liberal philosophies. People voiced rejection and, over time, voted for leaders who espoused smaller government and greater privatization. The new system protected the powerful and led to greater corruption. Bribes, kickbacks, and voter fraud were reported in all countries. Rathbone (2017) observes that this sequence is typical of many leaders. He opines that populist politicians eventually lead constituents to an authoritarian system by claiming projected changes to improve the political system are the "will of the people." The leader touts vague groups as his enemies (most often identified as foreigners or elites). Rathbone believes this approach eventually backfires when the populace realizes the corruption that leaves institutions (public and private) weak and a government in disarray.

LEARNING ACTIVITIES

1. Select one country within South America. Determine the type of government, structure, and points of access to address a health problem.

2. Identify what data you would need to take to policy makers to defend your position for change. How would you present imperfect or incomplete data?

3. List at least four stakeholders whom you could organize to assist you.

4. Develop responses to requests from officials for bribes.

CONCLUSION

A question arises: How can a person make a difference in a country in which healthcare is not a priority (usually noted by lack of funding), is inconsistently provided to the populace, is outdated, or is hampered by government structures and/or processes? Healthcare is provided in many ways and through many governmental and non-governmental venues. If health is a real determinant of the ability to function well in any society, then every society must bear responsibility for providing care so that the citizens will be healthy, safe, and productive. One person can begin by asking questions, building networks, and challenging the current healthcare system. Leadership requires persistence, persistence, persistence, to reach meaningful goals.

WEB RESOURCES

www.aihw.gov.au/reports/life-expectancy-death/deaths-in-australia/contents/multiple-causes-of-death

www.ama.com.au/ausmed/five-most-pressing-health-priorities-2014

www.aph.gov.au

www.australia.gov.au/about

www.australia.gov.au/information-and-services/health

www.avert.org/professionals/hiv-around-world/sub-saharan-africa/Nigeria

www.cdc.gov/nchs/products/databriefs/db293.html

www.indiancountrymedianetwork.com

REFERENCES

Artiga, S., Arguello, K., & Duckett, P. (2013). Health coverage and care for American Indians and Alaska natives *The Kaiser Family Foundation*. Retrieved from https://www.kff.org/disparities-policy/issue-brief/health-coverage-and-care-for-american-indians-and-alaska-natives

Avert. (2017). Men who have sex with men (MSM), HIV and AIDS. Retrieved from https://www.avert.org/professionals/hiv-social-issues/key-affected-populations/men-sex-men

BBC. (2016). What is India's caste system? Retrieved from http://www.bbc.com/news/world-asia-india-35650616

Brown, G. M. (2013). Nigerian political system: An analysis. *International Journal of Humanities and Social Science, 3*(10), 172–179.

Central Intelligence Agency. (2018). The world factbook: India. Retrieved from https://www.cia.gov/library/publications/the-world-factbook/geos/in.html

Constitution of Nigeria. (1999). Retrieved from http://www.nigeria-law.org/ConstitutionOfTheFederalRepublicOfNigeria.htm

Dhirag, A. B. (2017). The list of the world's 25 healthiest countries may surprise you. *CEO World Magazine*. Retrieved from http://ceoworld.biz/2017/04/19/list-worlds-25-healthiest-countries-may-surprise

Donatini, A. (2016). The Italian health care system. Retrieved from http://international.commonwealthfund.org/countries/italy

Gardner, J. (2015, December). Australian health system faces a "triple whammy," says KPMG health expert Mark Britnell. *The Sydney Morning Herald*. Retrieved from https://www.smh.com.au/business/the-economy/australian-health-system-faces-triple-whammy-says-kpmg-health-expert-mark-britnell-20151201-glcf5x.html

Gone, J., & Trimble, J. (2012). American Indian and Alaska Native mental health: diverse perspectives on enduring disparities. *Annual Review of Clinical Psychology, 8*, 131–160. doi:10.1146/annure-clinpsy-032511-143127

Gupta, I., & Bhatia, M. (2016). The Indian health care system profiles. Retrieved from www.international.commonwealthfund.org/countries/india

Harrison, C., Henderson, J., Miller, G., & Britt, H. (2017, March 9). The prevalence of diagnosing chronic conditions and multimorbidity in Australia: A method for estimating population prevalence from general practice patient encounter data. *PLOS ONE, 12*(3), e0172935. doi:10.1371/journal.pone.0172935

Health in South America. (2012). *Health situations, policy and systems overview. Organizacion Panamericana de la Salud.* Washington, DC: Pan American Health Organizacion and WHO.

Lu, W., & DelGiudice, V. (2017a). Italy's struggling economy has world's healthiest people. Retrieved from www.bloomberg.com/news/articles/2017-03-20/italy-s-struggling-economy-has-world-s-healthiest-people

Lu, W., & DelGiudice, V. (2017b, May 16). A tale of two economies. Retrieved from www.Economist.com/news/finance-and-economics/21651261-north-limps-ahead-southswoons-tale-two-economies

Macri, J. (2016). Australia's health system: Some issues and challenges. *Journal of Health and Medical Economics, 2016, 2,* 2. doi:10.21767/2471-9927.100015

McLuan, M., & Fiore, Q. (1968). *War and peace in the global village.* New York, NY: McGraw Hill.

Mercer, R. (2015). Policies, politics and the right to child health in South America. *BMJ Journal, 100*(51), S66–S69. doi:10.1136/archdischild-2013-305428

Mibeki digs in on AIDS. (2000, September 20). *BBC News.* 18:40. Retrieved from http://news.bbc.co.uk/2/hi/africa/934435.stm

Miroff, N. (Apr 16, 2017). Protests sweeping SouthAmerican show rising anti-government anger. *The Washington Post,* The Americas.

Moore, S.P., Soerjomataram, I., Green, A.C., Garvey, G., Martin, J., & Valery, P.C. (2016). Breast cancer diagnosis, patterns of care and burden of disease in Queensland, Australia (1998-2004): Does being Indigenous make a difference? *International Journal of Public Health, 61*(4), 435-542.

Mossialos, E., & Wenzel, M. (2015). International profiles of health care systems. Retrieved From www.commonwealthfund.org/~/media/files/publications/fund-report/2016/Jan/1857-mossialos-intl-profiles-2015-V7.pdf

National HIV/AIDS Stigma Reduction Strategy. (2017, May). Abuja, Nigeria: Cultural Business District. Nigeria now is free of Ebola. Retrieved from http://www.who.int/mediacentre/news/ebola/20-october-2014/en

Parliament of Australia. (n.d.). Retrieved from https://www.aph.gov.au/

Participant guide 2016-2018-Antarctic basics. Retrieved from https://www.usap.gov/USAPgov/travelAndDeployment/documents/ParticipantGuide_2016-18.pdf

Polio Global Eradication Initiative. (2017). Retrieved from www.polioeradication.org/this-world

Population Reference Bureau. (2002). Africa's political response to HIV/AIDS. Retrieved from http://www.prb.org/africaspoliticalresponsetohivaids

Rathbone, J. P. (2017, April 4). Old versus new is the real political divide in South American. *The Financial Times.* Retrieved from https://www.ft.com/content/ca001554-190b-11e7-9c35-0dd2cb31823a

Santevecchi, G. (2016). Living la dolce vita. *The Guardian.* Retrieved from https://www.theguardian.com/world/2006/jul/04/italy.lifeandhealth

Sarche, M., & Spicer, P. (2008). Poverty and health disparities for American Indians and Alaska Native children: Current knowledge and future prospects.

American Annals of NY Academy of Science, 1136, 126–136. doi:10.1196/ annals.1425.017

Sengupta, D. (2017, March). India ranks 148 in representation of women in government. Retrieved from http://www.newindianexpress.com/states/ tamil-nadu/2017/mar/17/india-ranks-148-in-representation-of-women -in-government-1582359.html

South American tribe found to have the healthiest hearts ever studied. (2017, March 18). *The Telegraph News.* Retrieved from https://www.telegraph.co.uk/ news/2017/03/18/south-american-tribe-found-have-healthiest-hearts-ever-studied

Taseer, A. (2016, October 12). India's eternal inequality. *New York Times.* Retrieved from https://www.nytimes.com/2016/10/13/opinion/indias -eternal-inequality.html

Ucheaga, D. N., & Hartwig, K. A. (2010). Religious leaders' response to AIDS in Nigeria. *Global Public Health, 5*(6), 611–625. doi:10.1080/17441690903463619

United Nations. (2015). World population prospects: Key findings and advance tables. Retrieved from https://esa.un.org/unpd/wpp/Publications/Files/ Key_Findings_WPP_2015.pdf

United States Antarctic Program. (n.d.). NSF Course Material. Retrieved from https://www.usap.gov/travelAndDeployment/contentHandler.cfm?id=1820

United States Antarctic Program. (2016–2018). Participant guide. Retrieved from https://www.usap.gov/USAPgov/travelAndDeployment/documents/ ParticipantGuide_2016-18.pdf

United States Census. (2010). About. Retrieved from https://www.census.gov/ topics/population/race/about.html

U.S. Department of State. (n.d.). Handbook of the Antarctic Treaty System. Retrieved from https://www.state.gov/e/oes/rls/rpts/ant/

Vu, L., Adebajo, S., Tun, W., Sheehy, M., Karlyn, A., Njab, J., ... Ahonsie, B. (2013). High HIV prevalence among men who have sex with men in Nigeria: Implications for combination therapy. *Journal of Acquired Immune Deficiency Syndromes, 63*(2), 221–227. doi:10.1097/QAI.0b013e31828e3e60

worldometers. (2017). Retrieved from http://www.worldometers.info/ world-population/south-america-population

Pandemics, Epidemics, and Outbreaks: Health Policy Research Priorities

Jessica Ellis
Mary de Chesnay
Genie E. Dorman
Adriana Caldwell

The purpose of this chapter is to highlight some of the health policy research related to recent pandemics and epidemics. A comprehensive review is beyond the scope of this book, but the authors think it is important to discuss some of the most recent global issues and the research methods used by policy makers. Providing examples of studies in these major areas gives an overview of the variety and depth of research methods that are used to study global health policy issues. However, any qualitative or quantitative methods that fit the research questions asked are appropriate.

PANDEMICS, EPIDEMICS, AND OUTBREAKS DEFINED

Sometimes, the amount of disease in a community increases above the expected level. *Epidemic* refers to a sudden increase in the number of cases of a disease above what is normally expected in that population in that area. *Outbreak* is used interchangeably with *epidemic*, but is often used for a more limited geographic area. *Pandemic* refers to an epidemic that has spread over several countries or continents, usually affecting a large number of people (Centers for Disease Control and Prevention [CDC], n.d.).

For example, a pandemic is a global outbreak of a disease when a new type of virus emerges and people have no immunity. The virus then spreads quickly and easily from person to person and causes serious illness worldwide, occurring simultaneously or in waves. HIV/AIDS is a good example of one of the most highly destructive pandemics in history. An epidemic is the rapid spread of a disease worldwide or highly localized with rapid spread from person to person. For example, SARS took the lives of more than 800,000 worldwide in 2003. An outbreak occurs when a disease occurs greater than expected within a community or region or during a specific season. In 2001, contamination of dialysis machines with perfluoroisobutylene caused unexpected deaths in six countries (World Health Organization [WHO], n.d.).

HIV/AIDS

GENERAL CALL FOR RESEARCH PRIORITIES

Global health policy is developed traditionally within countries as each nation responds to health issues affecting their populace. However, a new way of linking the development of policy with research is needed to address complex health problems that are truly global in nature. Jones, Clavier, and Potvin (2017) used methods of political science research to suggest a team approach in which various policy actors work together in an organized and interactive way rather than in stages of a policy cycle. They first conducted a state-of-the-art literature review to identify a framework for national strategies on global health policy.

In the United States, citizens have traditionally ranked national priorities over global priorities, chief among them being HIV/AIDS knowledge. Okamoto et al. (2011) surveyed 995 Americans (who were mostly white, married, and female) about their knowledge of HIV and their global health priorities and found that those with greater knowledge of HIV place greater emphasis on global health priorities.

Not surprisingly, past research efforts on HIV/AIDS have focused on epidemiological transmission and physiological responses and the result has been successful antiviral drug treatment (McGrath et al., 2014). As the state-of-the-art knowledge has expanded, researchers now address the need for understanding the effect of the disease on individuals. At the heart of this movement is the recognition by global health researchers that traditional anthropological or qualitative methods are most effective at eliciting the lived experience of HIV/AIDS (Nguyen, 2013).

Mazanderani and Paparini (2015) conducted 76 interviews with 35 people living with HIV/AIDS. Interviews lasted 1 to 2 hours, and one or two interviews were conducted in London over a span of 1 year. The sample included many immigrants from Africa, both heterosexual and homosexual. Their semistructured interviews were, for the most part, audiotaped and transcribed. Three major themes emerged from the data: normalization, biomedicalization, and discrimination. A gay British man described normalization as "living with HIV is better than living with cancer" as long as he managed his disease appropriately by taking meds and protected sex. The medicalization of their lives was described poignantly by a heterosexual woman from Zimbabwe who described depression and nightmares from her medications. A heterosexual man from Zimbabwe described how people shunned him in the belief that they would catch the disease by being close to him.

Although many people will not tell their stories in the belief that they do not matter, the authors assert that every story is significant. Policy makers need to be able to understand exactly how people's lives are affected by a disease that has lost much of its power to frighten, but that is by no means a relic of the past.

An international team from the United States, the United Kingdom, and South Africa collaborated with the World Health Organization (WHO) to identify research priorities for adolescent health in low- and middle-income countries. Nagata, Ferguson, and Ross (2016) recruited 142 experts who identified six health areas for priority research according to several criteria: descriptive epidemiology, interventions, discovery, development/testing, delivery, and policy. The highest health area for priority research was communicable diseases, particularly linking tuberculosis with HIV/AIDS.

REGIONAL ISSUES

Countries and regions have certainly studied HIV issues within their own borders. Canadians recognize that much research now takes place within an involved community. Guta et al. (2014) describe what they call citizen science or community-based research in which the community partners with the professionals to meet specific goals related to the topic that are not only important scientifically but also highly relevant to the affected community.

In the South Pacific, a number of countries have gained independence and are actively building their "nation-states" by contributing to global policy and programs about HIV/AIDS. In a recent study, an interdisciplinary research team found that global health programs not only focus on health but also have non-health-related outcomes in international relations, development, and unity (Kevany et al., 2015).

In Cartagena, Columbia, researchers conducted a qualitative study of patients, followed up by interviews with key policy makers. The findings revealed little cooperation with the church, barriers related to corruption, and lack of access to services (Djellouli & Quevedo-Gomez, 2015).

In resource-poor settings such as Malawi, models were borrowed from successful tuberculosis campaigns to increase the administration of antiretroviral therapy (ART). Malawi launched an innovation strategy of providing lifelong ART to pregnant women. The strategy was adopted by the WHO in its plan to end AIDS by 2030 (Harries, Ford, Jahn, Schouten, & Libamba, 2016).

Similarly, the Republic of Congo successfully combined tuberculosis and HIV programs to reverse its leading cause of death of HIV patients: tuberculosis. However, this resource-poor country lacks the support services to follow through adequately on the WHO recommendations, which are generic and do not necessarily reflect local culture factors (Linguissi et al., 2017).

INFLUENZA

Influenza epidemics are particularly challenging because the disease can strike anyone anywhere, even with vaccination because new strains evolve. However, it is possible to predict the most at-risk populations and develop policies for vaccination campaigns to target them. In a study conducted in the Phoenix metropolitan area, researchers found that they could localize clusters of outbreaks to target specific groups before the next outbreak (Kannan et al., 2016). They conducted a prospective observational surveillance study of 1,360 patients in which they mapped groups at risk. They then identified the densest cluster of patients and targeted this area for the next vaccination campaign.

Goldizen (2016) used international relations theory to study China's reversed position from isolation and resistance to active cooperation with international aid organizations during the SARS and avian flu epidemics. Using a series of case studies, the researcher concluded that it is critical to consider domestic policies when analyzing country-specific international relations during such emergencies.

We know that isolation of infected individuals is a highly effective way of controlling the spread of disease, but Liu et al. (2015) asked the question, "Which age groups should be singled out particularly?" They examined epidemiological data in south central China and found that isolating people between 25 and 59 was effective, but that isolating young children and older adults did not reduce their total attack rates. They concluded that this was not surprising given that the 25 to 59 age group was the largest population group, but warned that policy makers need to consider the cost–benefit ratio of isolating a large segment of the working population.

In another Chinese study, researchers conducted a household survey to examine implementation of the policy of free vaccinations to the elderly (Li et al., 2016; Lv et al., 2016). The government has long adhered to a policy of free vaccinations to poor elderly, but the study found that the policy favored poor higher-educated elderly in rural areas and suggested that more focus should be given to urban elderly populations.

TUBERCULOSIS

HOW GOVERNMENTS HANDLE TUBERCULOSIS OUTBREAKS

Tuberculosis (TB) is a disease caused by the bacteria *Mycobacterium tuberculosis* (MT). TB is often unnoticed for it is contagiously airborne through coughing and sneezing. Even though the bacteria usually affect the lungs, they can affect other parts of the body. TB is a deadly disease that affected 10.4 million people and led to 1.4 million deaths in 2015. Ranked as one of the leading deadliest epidemics in the world, TB infection is steadfastly rising, with 580,000 new cases of drug-resistant strains in 2015. The airborne transmittance makes tuberculosis so deadly because one could contract TB while inhaling the air of someone who has the disease. India, China, and Indonesia have the highest rates of TB followed by 19 other countries in Africa and the Middle East (TB Facts, 2018).

Tuberculosis control policy is developed differently within every country as they deal with their rate of TB and their populace. India has the largest TB outbreak in the world. Showing India's dire condition,

Verguet et al. (2014) stated there are "2 million active [TB] infections and 300,000 deaths from TB in India." To control such high rates, India devised evaluating TB cases through contact investigations. Contact investigations are a systematic process that identifies people exposed to someone with infectious TB disease, tests for infection of MT and TB disease, and provides them with treatment. Actively conducting contact investigations were hypothesized to reduce TB cases and implement early identification. Therefore, the study evaluated "the influence of screening household contacts possessing sputum smear-positive TB (viable TB bacteria) by implementing a procedure for contact investigation using healthcare staff and resources" (Khaparde et al., 2015). The rural, poor district of Rajnandgaon in Chhattisgarh State, India, was where the study was conducted. All households were visited and contacts were recorded. If any contact missed the first and second home visit, a slip was left with instructions for going to evaluations. To show more active engagement, phone calls were made after 1 week for contacts who failed to go to evaluation. Contacts with a sputum smear-positive contact were tested again. If symptoms persisted after 2 weeks, then further diagnosis continued with chest radiography examination and tuberculin skin test (Khaparde et al., 2015). The Indian government possessed national guidelines to treat TB; however, contact investigations helped an "additional 17 more TB cases" than average (Khaparde et al., 2015).

Despite every nation's guidelines for controlling TB, the TB burden still remains high because of economic cost. Most of the TB practitioners have private practices, which raise funds exponentially. Therefore, patients are compelled to pay out of pocket, making "medical cost the leading cause of high poverty rates" (Verguet et al., 2014). Another study found a majority, 25% of 41 households, of people in low/middle-income countries had to either borrow money or sell items to cover health cost. India's Universal Public Finance enables access to care that would be unaffordable otherwise, but it does not possess comprehensive coverage such as funds for transportation. Because of the high cost of TB treatment, China engaged in a new policy of implementing.

China has the world's second largest TB incidence after India. China's government partnered with the WHO and received funding from World Bank Loan and the Chinese Ministry for the project. The methodology included sending patients who were suspected of having TB for diagnosis by smear microscopy and radiography free of charge. Patients with TB were treated with free first-line drugs to remove financial barriers. Jia et al. tested the effectiveness of TB care according to national and local guidelines and whether free TB care was effectively implemented. TB diagnosis and treatment guidelines were examined to see whether TB care providers followed the guidelines. Next, a patient survey and interview was conducted to investigate spending funds. Even though TB prevalence was reduced to more than half, the hospitals did not follow national guidelines.

Africa has the third largest TB rate, and TB is the leading cause of death among HIV victims in Africa. High TB rates occur from TB transmission in healthcare facilities, and Africa's unique strain of mycobacterium is difficult to treat and costly. Therefore, every country is required by the WHO to report laws and statistics back to the organization. In Botswana, medically certified patients with the contagious disease is authorized for isolation until they are no longer infectious. South Africa has a constitution and guidelines controlling the handling of TB especially. Standards are set out to control TB in Section 2.6.2. Specific precautions are taken to prevent the spread of respiratory infection (South African Constitution, 1996). Every doctor is required to document TB, and South African National TB Management Guidelines calls for TB surveillance in healthcare workers. Zambia also has TB protection laws and guidelines. Under the Public Health Act, medical officers are required to receive reports of TB and employers report cases among employees and check up weekly on all TB cases and deaths. Overall, South Africa, Botswana, and Zambia all take exceptional precautions in reporting and controlling TB infection. Botswana has the policy to screen workers for TB and HIV. South Africa has a constitution with the universal right to healthcare services, whereas Zambia has a regulatory policy of specifically reporting TB. West Africa possesses similar discrepancies with TB and HIV much like Southern African countries. Another major dilemma with TB disease is that some strains of MT are becoming resistant to powerful first- and second-line drugs. Resistance intensifies the difficulty in controlling TB. Therefore, in these West African countries, multidrug-resistant (MDR) treatment is not totally accessible or effective. Gehre and her team (2016) wanted to show those West African countries that "drug-resistant TB is important in West African countries." Therefore, this will justify implementation of standardized (inter)national drug susceptibility testing (DST) ... and adequate MDR treatment programs across West Africa and prepare the region for new TB regimens for MDR-TB (Gehre et al., 2016). West African Network of Excellence for TB, AIDS, and Malaria (WANETAM) was founded with study sites all in Burkina Faso, Gambia, Ghana, Guinea-Bissau, Mali, Nigeria, Senegal, and Togo. Out of 1,568 TB isolates, 1,462 were collected.

The outcome of these numbers ended with 974 isolates (66%), which were included in the drug-resistant survey. Whereas 39% of the isolated bacteria showed resistance to some first-line drugs, there were no second-line resistance strains in the isolate, but 41 (21%) possessed developing strains resistant to second-line drugs. Retreatment patients were more than four times likely to be resistant to first-line drugs compared with new patients. Studies show resistance to first-line TB drugs is a major problem and resistance to second-line drugs is an emerging complication. For example, "Mali (59%) and the Nigerian study sites in Lagos (66%) and Ibadan (39%) had the highest percentages of MDR-TB" (Gehre, 2016). The studies found TB rates were higher than what the WHO predicted. For example, "Five out of nine and seven out of nine WANETAM sites were above the global TB prevalence average, and seven out of nine and eight out of nine WANETAM sites were above the estimated African MDR prevalence average." This study helped bring needed attention to the TB emergency of which the West African governments minimized the importance. More needs to be done in West Africa to combat the problem of MT resistance because the TB outbreak continues to worsen.

The Middle East ranks fourth on the list of the largest TB outbreaks. Even though Pakistan has the National TB Control Programme, which covers the policy of MDR-TB, the country acquired the same problem of controlling multidrug-resistant MT like in West Africa. MDR-TB is "man-made and develops during inappropriate TB treatment … and poor knowledge of patient towards therapy" (Javaid et al., 2016). Javaid studied the occurrence of TB either in the form of treatable TB or MDR-TB in household contacts. His team used a similar treatment as in the household contact investigation in India. MDR-TB patients were evaluated during home visits conducted by hospital representatives and then sputum tested. The productive ages (15–44 years) were the most affected. However, out of 235 sputum tests, 51 were positive for acid-fast bacilli, 184 were negative, and 218 contacts were only symptomatic. Results were low; however, this study brings awareness to the importance of early identification and diagnosis for prevention. Javaid and his team further justified this when they found that "screening household contacts in areas with high incidence of HIV-positive TB cases lead to the diagnosis of active infection up to nine-fold compared to passive endings." Thus, the importance of early screening is indisputable. An excellent study by Probandari evaluated how operational research (OR) can "influence TB policies, strategies that can enhance quality, effectiveness, or coverage of programs being done" (Probandari, 2016). The researchers studied how the Indonesian government handles TB control by dividing responsibilities between different levels of government. For example, the district government conducts basic management of TB control, such as drug distribution, lab supplies, and monitoring and supervising health facilities. The central government supervises standards related to TB and quality of TB drugs. The Tuberculosis Operational Research Group (TORG) formed by the National Tuberculosis Program has been conducting OR training since 2004. Thirty-three OR groups participated in the TORG and 31 groups conducted research. Interviews were conducted with results and recommendations of OR, follow-up actions, and the influence of OR on policy. OR has had 20 projects improve TB implementation, and 3 OR projects improved TB policy. Probandari's study found that "most OR projects contributed to TB policy and practice," and some innovated their policies because of the OR project. The United Kingdom would be the last country expected on a high-incidence TB chart; however, England experiences many immigrants from high-TB-rate countries moving into low-TB-rate areas.

TB cases increased continuously over the past few decades. For example, "out of 9000 cases in 2011, 74% came from foreigners" (O'Shea et al., 2014). An effective way of reducing TB rates is by screening patients. O'shea's study focuses on immigrants being screened for TB before entering the United Kingdom. The results showed the total number of TB cases declined in a year since migration. Preentry screening occurred in Britain as well as with Gurkha soldiers from Nepal. The United Kingdom screened for latent TB and worm infections common in soldiers using skin and blood tests. These tests were specific and effective in diagnosing latent TB, and the more specific results of the parasite were identified.

TB is also prevalent in children. A vaccine called Bacillus Calmette–Guérin (BCG) prevents severe TB from infecting children; however, it is not readily accessible to countries with low TB rates given its cost. The WHO produced three BCG vaccines (BCG Japan, Denmark, and Russia) in large amounts, yet the demand continues to grow higher. Kontturi et al. conducted a study on the availability of BCG vaccine across Europe. Kontturi et al.'s study shows 8 of 11 countries had BCG shortage and 7 of 8 changed immunization practices and policies. As of now, there is no current knowledge on national and global assessment of the impact of the BCG deficit on children with TB.

Overall, TB is a major problem in India, China, the Middle East, Indonesia, and the United Kingdom; however, each of these areas studied are controlling TB well. The affected countries recognize that it is a problem and enforce guidelines and regulations to reduce rates. In India, the government is handling TB well through contact investigations but health coverage needs to be improved. The Universal Public Finance program does not offer comprehensive coverage. TB is a tremendous problem in China, and China's government needs to become more involved in TB policy to effect a drastic change. The TB outbreak in Africa coupled with HIV heightens the outbreak problem. Despite this dual effect, the Southern African countries are effectively handling the outbreak of TB by enforcing laws and regulations to effectively control TB. Although the consequences of the TB burden in West Africa was undermined because the TB rate was higher than what WHO predicted, the WANETAM, fortunately, helped initiate TB research in West Africa and the conditions are expected to improve. In Pakistan, the TB outbreak is a growing problem but the government is handling it well by conducting active treatment in the form of screening and home visits. Indonesia is approaching TB well with its OR policy. The OR project established communication between OR groups and policymakers to ensure OR recommendations would last. TB is an emerging problem in England because of TB-infected immigrants, who intensify transmissions. The United Kingdom is administrating TB measures effectively with preentry screenings. Screening for TB early and conducting contact investigation leads to the early identification, diagnosis, and treatment. BCG has the potential to save many more lives from TB, but the WHO needs to devise a plan for this problem.

MATERNAL MORBIDITY AND MORTALITY

Reducing maternal morbidity and mortality is a major global health challenge. Worldwide, at least one woman dies every 2 minutes from complications in pregnancy or childbirth (Lassi et al., 2016; Makanga, Schuurman, von Dadelszen, & Firoz, 2016). The WHO estimates that every day approximately 830 women die from preventable causes related to pregnancy. In 2015, 303,000 women died from complications during pregnancy or childbirth. We begin to see the magnitude of the problem when we look at the number of pregnancies and births occurring yearly. Each year 210 million women become pregnant, and 140 million newborn babies are delivered (Graham et al., 2016). Maternal mortality rates are higher among women who live in rural areas, and poor women and adolescents face a higher risk of complications and death as a result of pregnancy than do other women (WHO, 2016).

Maternal health is the health of women during pregnancy, childbirth, and the postpartum period (WHO, n.d.). *Maternal mortality,* or maternal death, is the death of women while pregnant or within 42 days of termination of pregnancy, irrespective of the duration and site of the pregnancy, from any cause related to the pregnancy, but not from accidental causes. Maternal mortality rates are measured by the maternal mortality ratio (per 100,000 live births). Live birth refers to the complete expulsion or extraction of the products of conception, which after separation show evidence of life (e.g., breathing and heartbeat). *Maternal morbidity* refers to conditions that are attributed to or aggravated by pregnancy and childbirth that have a negative impact on a woman's well-being. Maternal morbidity is harder to track than maternal mortality; estimates suggest that for every woman who dies, 20 to 30 women suffer from complications related to childbirth. The complications of maternal morbidity can be long term and devastating, resulting in infertility or damage to reproductive organs (Makanga et al., 2016).

Major causes of morbidity and mortality include hemorrhage, infection, high blood pressure, unsafe abortion, and obstructed labor (WHO, 2016). Less than 1% of maternal deaths occur in developed countries. Therefore, most maternal deaths occur in low- to middle-income countries, with the highest number occurring in sub-Saharan Africa and Southeast Asia.

WORLDWIDE MATERNAL HEALTH GOALS

Millennium Development Goals

The Millennium Development Goals (MDG) were created by the United Nations in 2000 as a global partnership to reduce extreme poverty (WHO, 2015). MDG 5: Improve Maternal Health was specifically designed to reduce the global maternal mortally rates and to provide access to reproductive health. Globally, it is estimated 289,000 women died during childbirth in 2013, which was a decline of approximately 45% from the level seen in 1990. Most women died because they had no access to skilled routine or emergency care. Since 1990, some countries in Asia and Northern Africa have reduced the maternal mortality rates by more than half.

Many countries were not successful in reaching MDG 5 because of many factors (WHO, 2015). A lack of access to care during pregnancy and childbirth, a shortage of trained healthcare workers, and poor access to contraceptive services were significant constraints noted for not attaining the maternal health–related MDG targets set forth by many countries. Providing adequate access to care can be complicated by both geography and infrastructure in many African and Asian countries. Areas lack infrastructure from roads to hospitals. A shortage of healthcare workers is seen globally due to uneven distribution of the healthcare workforce. For example, Asia has half of the world population, but only has access to 30% of the healthcare workforce. The shortage of emergency obstetric care and surgical services in low- to middle-income countries has attracted government attention and a closer look at the allocation of resources worldwide. Globally, over 10% of women do not have access to or are not using an effective method of contraception. It has been estimated that meeting the needs for contraception could reduce the number of maternal deaths by almost a third.

Sustainable Development Goals

The newly developed Sustainable Development Goals (SDG) consist of 17 goals with 169 target measures (United Nations, n.d.). The health of women and girls will be most affected by Goal 3—ensure healthy lives and promote well-being for all at all stages. This goal aims at improving maternal health in two different ways: (1) to reduce the maternal mortality ratio to less than 70 per 100,000 live births and (2) to ensure universal access to sexual and reproductive healthcare services for family planning, information and education, and the integration of reproductive health into national strategies and programs.

STRATEGIES TO IMPROVE MATERNAL HEALTH

The WHO (2015) has five key working areas that include policy and programs focused in the following areas: (1) strengthening health systems by promoting policies and interventions that work within each regional system; (2) monitoring and evaluating the burden of poor maternal health; (3) building effective partnerships that make the best use of scarce resources and reduce duplication of services; (4) advocating for investment in maternal health by highlighting the economic benefits and emphasizing maternal mortality as a human rights issue; and, finally, (5) coordinating research with wide-scale applications that focus on improving maternal health in pregnancy and the postpartum period.

A large-cluster, randomized, controlled trial is underway in Uttar Pradesh, India, to test the effectiveness of the WHO Safe Childbirth Checklist (Semrau et al., 2016). If effective, the WHO Safe Childbirth Checklist could be a powerful tool in strengthening health-related facility interventions, improving the quality of care, and reducing preventable harm to women and newborns. The impact of the intervention could potentially affect millions of lives annually.

Countries that have been successful in achieving progress toward global maternal health goals show consistent and coordinated efforts in policy and programming across health and other sectors such as investing in the girl child's educations, water sanitization, hygiene, reducing poverty, nutrition and food security, and infrastructure development (Ahmed et al., 2016). Ahmed et al. (2016) reports approaches used successfully by countries such as Cambodia, Rwanda, Lao People's Democratic Republic, Nepal, Peru, China, and Ethiopia have reduced the maternal mortality ratio between the years 1990 and 2015 by more than 5% annually.

EBOLA-MARBURG

Ebola virus disease (EVD) and Marburg are both hemorrhagic fevers that are acute viral diseases leading to severe illness and even death (National Institute of Health [NIH], 2016). According to the National Institute of Health (NIH), the infections typically affect multiple body systems and organs and are often accompanied by hemorrhage (bleeding). The NIH reports that once the virus is transmitted from an animal host to a human, it can then spread through person-to-person contact. Fatality rates are defined by the *case fatality rate* (CFR), which is the proportion of deaths within a designated population of "cases" (people with the medical condition) over the course of the disease. The fatality rates are similar for Ebola and Marburg, with both having an average fatality rate of around 50% and with case fatality rates ranging from 25% to 90% in recent outbreaks (WHO, 2017). Because of the recent Ebola outbreaks and the availability of literature on the topic, Ebola will be the focus of discussion in the remainder of this section.

RECENT EBOLA OUTBREAKS

West Africa recently experienced the largest outbreak of Ebola ever recorded, overwhelming the capacity of local health systems and the international community in providing needed treatment and isolation to prevent the spread of the disease (Levine et al., 2015). Levine et al. (2015) constructed an Ebola prediction score using retrospective patient data. The group identified six variables that were independently predictive for laboratory-confirmed Ebola including skin contact, diarrhea, loss of appetite, muscle pains, difficulty swallowing, and absence of abdominal cramping. Patients with higher Ebola prediction score had higher likelihoods of laboratory-confirmed Ebola virus disease. The Ebola prediction score can be used by clinics for risk stratification in patients with suspected Ebola virus disease. This tool can be used to group patients in isolation or as a triage tool when patient numbers overwhelm available capacity.

Many hospitals were challenged with containing a highly infectious disease during the 2014 to 2105 Ebola outbreak. To study hospital preparation for the potential emergence of a highly contagious disease, Broom, Broom, and Bowden (2017) conducted structured interviews with 21 healthcare providers in Australian hospitals. These interviews focused on participant views regarding information, training, and preparedness, to inform future outbreak preparedness training. Three key themes in relationship to Ebola preparedness planning are (1) the impact of high volumes of inconsistent information in shaping trust in authority, (2) barriers to engagement in training, including the perceived relative risk Ebola presented, and (3) practical and environmental impediments to preparedness (Broom, Broom, & Bowden, 2017). Understanding that risk and trust overlap with communication, preparedness, and environmental logistics was crucial to effective preparation and management of a highly contagious outbreak such as Ebola.

PUBLIC PERCEPTIONS OF RISK REGARDING EBOLA

Risk and public perceptions of trust with the media were explored in two studies, where the moderate likelihood that a person might exhibit symptoms after a 21-day exposure to Ebola was given to participants in two different ways (Johnson & Slovic, 2015). One study examined the effects of giving quantitative data estimates of symptoms being present after a 21-day exposure to Ebola ($n = 1,413$), and the other study used a mock news story where Ebola was contracted after 21 days of exposure ($n = 425$). Both studies revealed that perceived risk increased and trust declined when people learned of post-21-day symptoms. The results of the studies reported by Johnson and Slovic (2015) suggest public health official should give all the facts, including unpleasant ones, early in the course of the epidemic to increase public trust in media reporting.

THE ROLE OF EBOLA POLICY DIALOGUES

Policy dialogues are recognized as an important part of global policy making. Interactive and innovative policy dialogue models were applied in different contexts related to the Ebola outbreaks (Nabyonga-Orem, Gebrikidane, & Mwisongo, 2016). Nabyonga-Orem et al. (2016) reported the results from an exploratory study from Liberia in which the role of context was highlighted as influencing stakeholders in policy making. The context for the policy dialogues in Liberia is set against the backdrop of Liberia being a postwar country, highly donor dependent, and in recovery from a catastrophic Ebola outbreak. In 16 interviews with key informants, both before and after the Ebola crisis, the context was reported as being instrumental in shaping the dialogues, including issues of focus, requirements for participation, and the decisions that were needed. Policy dialogues are a platform for policy discussion and decisions in Liberia. The process of including context was recognized and appreciated in contributing to the success of the negations during and after the Ebola outbreak.

STRATEGIES TO PREVENT FUTURE EBOLA OUTBREAKS

The WHO continues to track the evolving Ebola and Marburg infectious disease situations, sound the alarm when needed, share experiences, and mount the appropriate response needed to protect the population from the consequences of a subsequent outbreak (WHO, 2017). Good outbreak control relies on applying interventions including community engagement, case management, surveillance and contact tracing, a good laboratory service, and support and training for safe burial practices. Raising awareness of risk factors for infection as well as protective measures such as vaccination, through community engagement, can be an effective way for individuals to reduce transmission and prevent future outbreaks. Risk awareness education should focus on reducing the risk of animal-to-human transmission, human-to-human transmission, and possible sexual transmission and on outbreak containment measures. Examples of outbreak containment measures are a prompt and safe burial of the dead, identifying people who had contact with the infected person, appropriate monitoring (21 days or longer), the importance of separating the sick from the healthy to prevent future spread, the need for good hygiene, and maintaining a clean environment.

SUMMARY

This chapter has been a brief presentation of some of the policy-related research around major disease outbreaks, epidemics, and pandemics of recent years. HIV/AIDS policy-related research is being addressed at all levels, including global and regional levels. Using a variety of research strategies, new emerging knowledge is being gained regarding the lived experience of individuals who are HIV positive. These research strategies have included qualitative interviews with people who are living with HIV, community-based research, and semistructured interviews with policy makers. In addition, research proprieties are being developed for research-ing the experiences of adolescent health with regard to HIV/AIDS. New policy implementation strategies have linked HIV and tuberculosis care in low-income countries.

Policy research related to minimizing the effects of influenza is difficult because influenza outbreaks are unpredictable and can occur anywhere at any time. The strategy of mapping has been used with some success to target specific groups before a localized outbreak. For example, research in Asia has shown isolation can be effective in reducing the spread of influenza. However, an outbreak may still greatly affect large numbers of working individuals. Offering free vaccines to high-risk targeted groups such as the elderly living in an urban area is another strategy that has been shown to be effective in reducing the spread of influenza. Tuberculosis continues to be a major problem in many coun-tries. The use of early screening, screening on entry to a country, and contact investigation have been shown to lead to overall lower rates of TB in high-risk countries.

In summary, it is evident that a variety of research methodologies are used to study country-specific policies regarding health and disease as well as the effects these policies and their implementation have on the impact of disease on the population.

ACKNOWLEDGMENTS

The authors are grateful to three nurse practitioner students who assisted with the literature review for this chapter: Giovanni Lopez, Sandeep Singhal, and Pinnakin Patel.

REFERENCES

Ahmed, S. M., Rawal, L. B., Chowdhury, S. A., Murray, J., Arscott-Mills, S., Jack, S., & Kuruvilla, S. (2016). Cross-country analysis of strategies for achieving progress towards global goals for women's and children's health. *Bull World Health Organ, 94*(5), 351–361. doi:10.2471/blt.15.168450

Broom, J., Broom, A., & Bowden, V. (2017). Ebola outbreak preparedness planning: A qualitative study of clinicians' experiences. *Public Health, 143*, 103–108. doi:10.1016/j.puhe.2016.11.008

Centers for Disease Control and Prevention. (n.d.). Principles of epidemiology in public health practice (3rd ed.). Retrieved from https://www.cdc.gov/OPHSS/CSELS/DSEPD/SS1978/Lesson1/Section11.html#_ref51

Djellouli, N., & Quevedo-Gomex, M. (2015). Challenges to successful implementation of HIV/AIDS-related policies in Cartagena, Columbia. *Social Sciences and Medicine, 33*, 36–44. doi:10.1016/j.socscimed.2015.03.048

Gehre, F., Otu, J., Kendall, L., Forson, A., Kwara, A., Kudzawu, S., ... Antonio, M. (2016). The emerging threat of pre-extensively drug-resistant tuberculosis in West Africa: Preparing for large-scale tuberculosis research and drug resistance surveillance. *BMC Medicine, 14*(1), 160. doi:10.1186/s12916-016-0704-5

Goldizen, C. (2016). From SARS to avian influenza: The role of international factors in China's approach to infectious disease control. *Annals of Global Health, 82*(1), 180–188. doi:10.1016/j.aogh.2016.01.024

Graham, W., Woodd, S., Byass, P., Filippi, V., Gon, G., Virgo, S., & Singh, S. (2016). Diversity and divergence: The dynamic burden of poor maternal health. *Lancet, 388*(10056), 2164–2175. doi:10.1016/s0140-6736(16)31533-1

Guta, A., Strike, C., Flicker, S., Murray, S., Upshur, R., & Myers, T. (2016). Governing through community-based research: Lessons from the Canadian HIV research sector. *Social Science and Medicine, 123*, 250–261. doi:10.1016/j.socscimed.2014.07.028

Harries, A., Ford, N., Jahn, A., Schouten, E., & Libamba, E. (2016). Act local, think global: How the Malawi experience of scaling up antiretroviral treatment has informed global policy. *BMC Public Health, 16*, 938. doi:10.1186/s12889-016-3620-x

Javaid, A., Khan, M. A., Khan, M. A., Mehreen, S., Basit, A., Khan, R. A., ... Ullah, U. (2016). Screening outcomes of household contacts of multidrug-resistant tuberculosis patients in Peshawar, Pakistan. *Asian Pacific Journal of Tropical Medicine, 9*(9), 909–912. doi:10.1016/j.apjtm.2016.07.017

Jia, X., Chen, J., Zhang, S., Dai, B., Long, Q., & Tang, S. (2016). Implementing a "free" tuberculosis (TB) care policy under the integrated model in Jiangsu, China: Practices and costs in the real world. *Infectious Diseases of Poverty, 5,* 1–8. doi:10.1186/s40249-016-0099-8

Johnson, B. B., & Slovic, P. (2015). Fearing or fearsome Ebola communication? Keeping the public in the dark about possible post-21-day symptoms and infectiousness could backfire. *Health and Risk Society, 17*(5–6), 458–471. doi:10.1080/13698575.2015.1113237

Jones, C., Clavier, C., & Potvin, L. (2017). Adapting public policy theory for public health research: A framework to understand the development of national policies on global health. *Social Science and Medicine, 177,* 69–77. doi:10.1016/j.socscimed.2017.01.048

Kannan, V., Hodgson, N., Lau, A., Goodin, K., Dugas, A., & LoVecchio, F. (2016). Geolocalization of influenza outbreak within an acute care population: A layered surveillance approach. *Annals of Emergency Medicine, 68*(5), 618–626. doi:10.1016/j.annemergmed.2016.07.025

Kevany, S., Gildea, A., Garae, C., Moa, S., & Lautusi, A. (2015). Global health diplomacy, national integration, and regional development through the monitoring and evaluation of HIV/AIDS programs in Papua New Guinea, Vanuatu, and Samoa. *International Journal of Health Policy Management, 4*(6), 337–341. doi:10.15171/ijhpm.2015.89

Khaparde, K., Jethani, P., Dewan, P., Nair, S., Deshpande, R., Satyanarayana, S., … Moonan. P. (2015). Evaluation of TB case finding through systematic contact investigation, Chhattisgarh, India. *Tuberculosis Research and Treatment, 2015.* doi:10.1155/2015/670167

Kontturi, A., Santiago, B., Tebruegge, M., von Both, U., Salo, E., & Ritz, N. (2016). The impact of Bacille Calmette-Guerin shortage on immunisation practice and policies in Europe: A Paediatric Tuberculosis Network European Trials Group (Ptbnet) survey. *Tuberculosis, 101,* 126–129. doi:10.1016/j.tube.2016.08.005

Lassi, Z. S., Musavi, N. B., Maliqi, B., Mansoor, N., de Francisco, A., Toure, K., & Bhutta, Z. A. (2016). Systematic review on human resources for health interventions to improve maternal health outcomes: Evidence from low- and middle-income countries. *Human Resources in Health, 14,* 10. doi:10.1186/s12960-016-0106-y

Levine, A. C., Shetty, P. P., Burbach, R., Cheemalapati, S., Glavis-Bloom, J., Wiskel, T., & Kesselly, J. K. (2015). Derivation and internal validation of the Ebola Prediction Score for risk stratification of patients with suspected Ebola virus disease. *Annals in Emergency Medicine, 66*(3), 285–293.e281. doi:10.1016/j.annemergmed.2015.03.011

Li, T., Lv, M., Lei, T., Wu, J., Pang, X., Deng, Y., & Xie, Z. (2016). Who benefits most from influenza vaccination policy: A study among the elderly in Beijing, China. *International Journal for Equity in Health, 15*, 45. doi:10.1186/s12939-016-0332-x

Linguissi, L., Gwom, L., Nkenfou, C., Batess, M., Petersen, E., Zumla, A., & Ntoumi, F. (2017). Health systems in Republic of Congo: Challenges and opportunities for implementing tuberculosis and HIV collaborative service, research and training activities. *International Journal of Infectious Diseases, 56*, 62–67. doi:10.1016/j.ijid.2016.10.012

Liu, R., Leung, R., Chen, T., Zhang, X., Chen, F., Chen, S., & Zhao, Z. (2015). The effectiveness of age-specific isolation policies on epidemics of influenza A (H1N1) in a large city in south central China. *PLOS One, 10*(7), e0132588. doi:10.1371/journal.pone.0132588

Lv, M., Fang, R, Wu, J., Pang, X., Deng, Y., Lei, T., & Xie, Z. (2016). The free vaccination policy in Beijing, China: The vaccine coverage and its associated factors. *Vaccine, 34*, 2135–2140. doi:10.1016/j.vaccine.2016.02.032

Makanga, P. T., Schuurman, N., von Dadelszen, P., & Firoz, T. (2016). A scoping review of geographic information systems in maternal health. *International Journal of Gynaecology and Obstetrics, 134*(1), 13–17. doi:10.1016/j.ijgo.2015.11.022

Mazanderani, F., & Paparini, S. (2015). The stories we tell: Qualitative research interviews, talking technologies, and the normalization of life with HIV. *Social Science and Medicine, 131*, 66–73. doi:10.1016/j.socscimed.2015.02.041

McGrath, J., Winchester, M., Kaawi-Mafigiri, D., Walakira, E., Namitibwa, F., Birungi, J., ... Rwabukwali, C. (2014). Challenging the paradigm: Anthropological perspectives on HIV as a chronic disease. *Medical Anthropology, 33*(4), 303–317. doi:10.1080/01459740.2014.892483

Nabyonga-Orem, J., Gebrikidane, M., & Mwisongo, A. (2016). Assessing policy dialogues and the role of context: Liberian case study before and during the Ebola outbreak. *BMC Health Services Research, 16*(Suppl 4), 219. doi:10.1186/s12913-016-1454-y

Nagata, J., Ferguson, B., & Ross, D. (2016). Research priorities for eight areas of adolescent health in low- and middle-income countries. *Journal of Adolescent Health, 59*(1), 50–60. doi:10.1016/j.jadohealth.2016.03.016

National Institute of Health. (2016). Ebola and Marburg. Retrieved from https://www.niaid.nih.gov/diseases-conditions/ebola-marburg

Nguyen, V. (2013). Counseling against HIV in Africa: A genealogy of confessional technologies. *Culture of Health and Sex, 15*(4), S440–S452. doi:10.1080/13691058.2013.809146

Okamoto, J., Buffington, S., Cloum, H., Mendenhalf, B., Toboni, M., & Valente, T. (2011). The influence of health knowledge in shaping political priorities: Examining HIV/AIDS knowledge and knowledge about global health and domestic policies. *Global Public Health, 6*(8), 830–842. doi:10.1080/17441 692.2010.551517

O'Shea, M. K., Fletcher, T. E., Tupper, D., Ross, D., & Wilson, D. (2014). Screening for latent tuberculosis and gastrointestinal parasite infections in Gurkha recruits: Research driving policy change. 180-82. *Journal of the Royal Army Medical Corps, 160*(2), 108–182. doi: 10.1136/jramc-2014-000259.

Probandari, A., Widjanarko, B., Mahendradhata, Y., Sanjoto, H., Cerisha, A., Nungky, S., … Alisjahbana, B. (2016). The path to impact of operational research on tuberculosis control policies and practices in Indonesia. *Global Health Action, 9.* doi: 10.3402/gha.v9.29866.

Semrau, K. E., Hirschhorn, L. R., Kodkany, B., Spector, J. M., Tuller, D. E., King, G., & Gawande, A. A. (2016). The effectiveness of the WHO Safe Childbirth Checklist program in reducing severe maternal, fetal, and newborn harm in Uttar Pradesh, India: Study protocol for a matched-pair, cluster-randomized controlled trial. *Trials, 17*(1), 576. doi:10.1186/s13063-016-1673-x

TB Facts. (2018). Retrieved from https://www.tbfacts.org/countries-tb/

United Nations. (n.d.). Health—United Nations sustainable development. Retrieved from http://www.un.org/sustainabledevelopment/health

Verani, A. R., Emerson, C. N., Lederer, P., Lipke, G., Kapata, N., Lanje, S., … Miller, B. (2016).The role of the law in reducing tuberculosis transmission in Botswana, South Africa and Zambia. *Bulletin of the World Health Organization, 94*(6), 415–423. doi: 10.2471/BLT.15.156927

Verguet, S., Laxminarayan, R., & Jamison, D. T. (2014). Universal public finance of tuberculosis treatment in India: An extended cost-effectiveness analysis. *Health Economics, 24*(3), 318–332. doi: 10.1002/hec.3019

World Health Organization. (n.d.). Maternal mortality ratio. Retrieved from http://www.who.int/healthinfo/statistics/indmaternalmortality/en

World Health Organization. (2015). MGD 5: Improve maternal health. Retrieved from http://www.who.int/topics/millennium_development_goals/maternal_health/en

World Health Organization. (2016). Maternal mortality—Fact sheet. Retrieved from http://www.who.int/mediacentre/factsheets/fs348/en

World Health Organization. (2017). Ebola virus disease—Fact sheet. Retrieved from http://www.who.int/mediacentre/factsheets/fs103/en

Healthcare Policy: Funding for Immigrants and Refugees

Brenda Brown

Healthcare costs and funding in the United States is an issue of serious magnitude. The United States has some of the most advanced healthcare services, technology, medications, and research in the Western world but spends more of its gross domestic product (GDP) on health-related matters than any other industrialized nation. Furthermore, healthcare costs in the United States are the highest globally, about 40% more per capita than other industrialized countries. Millions of individuals are uninsured or underinsured, including a large number of immigrants and refugees (Squires & Anderson, 2015). The Patient Protection and Affordable Healthcare Act of 2010 contains significant reforms to make healthcare coverage more affordable and healthcare services easier to access (HealthCare.gov, 2013). The legislation has sparked many debates about the role of government in providing healthcare, and people on both sides of the issue have strong feelings about whether immigrants and refugees deserve access to healthcare, especially healthcare funded by the government.

The scope of this paper is to explore policies related to healthcare funding for immigrants and refugees, the consequences of not providing healthcare, and current legislation addressing the topic. Furthermore, the author discusses healthcare needs, access, and funding for a specific group of immigrants and refugees—Afghan women in the greater Atlanta area.

Moreover, the author discusses the criteria that differentiate refugees, documented immigrants, and undocumented immigrants. A brief overview of the history of U.S. immigration legislation as well as legislation related to healthcare issues of refugees and immigrants is examined. Finally, the author recounts specific field work undertaken to explore healthcare legislation and services to immigrants and refugees in the state of Georgia, with a particular interest in the population of Afghan women.

IMMIGRANTS AND REFUGEES: WHO ARE THEY?

Immigrants are people from other countries who come to the United States to live and generally plan to become citizens. Documented (legal) immigrants have usually been invited by the United States to work, live, or reunite with family. Undocumented (illegal) immigrants have come without proper documentation such as visas, green cards, work permits (State of Georgia, n.d.).

Refugees are individuals or families who are fleeing their native country and coming to the United States because they are facing political unrest, war, persecution, or natural disasters. Refugees must prove that danger or persecution does exist in their native country and that they are facing a real and immediate threat to safety and wellbeing (Immigration Policy Center, 2013; State of Georgia, n.d.).

However, applying for and receiving immigration or refugee status is not an easy undertaking. A number of issues lead to delays in obtaining legal residency in the United States. Extensive paperwork must be completed and specific criteria met for each classification. For example, an individual coming as a student versus one coming as part of a family reunification program would have to fulfill different criteria and complete a different application process. Adding to the complicated process is the involvement of multiple federal and state agencies, with each agency having its own policies. Long wait times for processing of applications is another issue, and if the application is incorrect, then the individual must resubmit and start the process again (Immigration Policy Center, 2013; State of Georgia Refugee Health Guideline Manual, n.d.). Finally, language barriers are another roadblock to applying for refugee/immigration status. Individuals must find someone who can and will provide interpretation of the forms and any spoken instructions (Edberg, Cleary, & Vyas, 2011).

HISTORY OF IMMIGRATION LEGISLATION

An extensive discussion of all U.S. immigrant and refugee legislation is beyond the scope of this paper, but some grasp of major policies is necessary as a foundation for comprehending healthcare legislation. Legislation directly addressing immigration has been in place since 1790 when a law was passed requiring a residency of 2 years in the United States before a person could become naturalized.

The next major law passed was the Steerage Act of 1819, which mandated that all U.S. ships would report immigrants in their manifests. In 1882, the Chinese Exclusion Act was passed, which suspended the immigration of Chinese laborers to the United States and barred any Chinese from becoming naturalized citizens. Additionally, this law allowed for the deportation of any Chinese immigrants in the country illegally (Ewing, 2012; Fix & Passel, 1994).

The Immigration Act of 1891 was the first national comprehensive law to control immigration. Under this law, the Bureau of Immigration was established as part of the Treasury Department, and again, any illegal alien was to be deported. The Immigration and Naturalization Act was initiated in 1924 and revised in 1952. These laws set limits on the numbers of immigrants and geographic locations from which they could enter the United States. Northern and Western Europeans were the favored populations for immigration. The Border Patrol was established under the provisions of the 1924 law, and the 1952 revision mandated a quota for immigrants who had skills greatly needed in the Unites States (Ewing, 2012; Fix & Passel, 1994).

Several immigration laws were instituted during the 1980s. The Refugee Act (1980) established specific criteria for this immigrant population and was the first legislation to establish a system for allowing refugees into the country and for categorizing them. A domestic resettlement program was also a section of this law. The Immigration Reform and Control Act (IRCA) of 1985 sanctioned a fee for employers who knowingly hired, recruited, or referred any illegal alien. Additional sections of this law created programs for the legalization of immigrants and increased enforcement at the borders. A $4 billion State Legalization Impact Assistance Grant Program was created under this law (Pandey & Kagotho, 2010; Viladrich, 2012).

The Immigration Act of 1990 increased the upper limit for legal immigrants by 40% and tripled the maximum number of employment-based immigrants. Furthermore, it created a diversity admissions category and established a temporary protected status for immigrants in the United States who were jeopardized by armed conflict or natural disasters in their native countries.

The final legislation discussed here is the Illegal Immigration Reform and Immigrant Responsibility Act of 1996. Under this law, U.S. citizens faced increased penalties for alien smuggling and document fraud and undocumented immigrants faced an expedited removal from the country. It also barred unlawfully present immigrants from re-entry for longer periods of time and capped income requirements for immigrant sponsors at 125% of federal poverty level (Ewing, 2012; Fix & Passel, 1994).

HEALTHCARE LEGISLATION

The literature review was accomplished by entering the phrase "U.S. healthcare legislation and immigrants" into the search engine, which yielded 27,544 hits. The author then focused on literature that had one of the following three central themes: how legislation has impacted healthcare services and funding for immigrants and refugees, comparisons of native-born citizen and immigrant/refugee use of healthcare services, and what amount of healthcare costs can be attributed to immigrants and refugees.

Since refugees have fled their native countries because of dangers and have been granted asylum by the United States, they are eligible for the Refugee Cash Assistance (RCA) and Refugee Medical Assistance (RMA) programs. These programs are supported 100% by federal funding and are available for 8 to 12 months from the date individuals first qualify for refugee status. Two programs offer financial and healthcare resources for refugees—Temporary Assistance for Needy Families (TANF) and Medicaid, provide healthcare coverage for families with minor children (Burr, Gerst, Kwan, & Mutchler, 2009; J. Mena, personal communication, April 16, 2013; Refugee Health Technical Support Center, 2011).

Immigrants, on the contrary, have no guaranteed access to healthcare funding or services. Some states and cities may provide limited benefits or individuals may have access to neighborhood healthcare and/or indigent clinics, which offer services regardless of immigrant status or income. However, for most immigrants, healthcare is a luxury and thus they live without it and hope for the best.

KEY HEALTHCARE LEGISLATION

One federal policy that influenced immigrants' access to healthcare was the Emergency Medical Treatment and Active Labor Act (EMTALA) of 1986. A key provision within EMTALA mandated that every patient who presented to the emergency department (ED) of a hospital that received Medicare funding must be granted appropriate treatment or stabilization before being discharged home or transferred to another facility regardless of the ability to pay (American College of Physicians, 2011; Gusmano, 2012; Tavis, 2010). This law opened a door for those who had previously been unable to afford healthcare services. The unfortunate outcome to this law was the influx of patients with nonemergent conditions, which created heavy burdens for hospitals and healthcare professionals.

The state of California submitted a bill in 1994, named Proposition 187, which denied access to many public services to undocumented immigrants, including education and healthcare. This proposition was declared unconstitutional; however, it had the effect of heightening anti-immigrant sentiments across the United States.

A key legislative act in 1996, the Personal Responsibility Work Opportunity Reconciliation Act (PRWORA), mandated that legal immigrants had to reside in the United States for a minimum of 5 years in order to be eligible for citizenship and federally funded healthcare coverage. The viewpoint of the legislators behind this law was that healthcare was a responsibility, not a right. Thus, thousands of refugees and legal immigrants lost healthcare coverage. Some states offered emergency Medicaid or granted other benefits to these people, but for the most part, healthcare coverage was non-existent. The result of this law was that immigrants began using EDs for primary care under the EMTALA and state healthcare costs increased significantly (Burr et al., 2009; Tavis, 2010; Viladrich, 2012).

The Deficit Reduction Act of 2005 required that everyone applying for or renewing Medicaid had to show proof of U.S. citizenship (Centers for Medicare and Medicaid Services, 2018). In 2006, the state of Massachusetts established An Act Providing Access to Affordable, Quality, and Accountable Healthcare, which meant that almost all citizens had some form of healthcare coverage. However, this act was revoked in 2009, leaving approximately 8,000 legal immigrants without healthcare coverage. The state of New Jersey enacted similar legislation in 2010, which impacted about 12,000 legal immigrants (Baiden, 2010; Tavis, 2010).

FINDINGS AND ANALYSIS

The literature review carried a theme of myths and facts about healthcare use by and the costs attributed to the immigrants, both legal and illegal. For this section of the paper, the author compares these myths and facts to provide an argument for the provision of healthcare to immigrants. Additionally, the author found that the myths had become part of her way of thinking about immigrants and appreciated the facts that helped to change this thinking.

MYTHS AND FACTS

One of the first myths noted in the literature is the belief that immigrants come just to get all they can for free. Many U.S. citizens feel that immigrants are living off of tax money and contributing nothing to society. The fact is that immigrants come to have a better life and to give their children a better chance. Most immigrants are fleeing extreme poverty, war, and oppression. They may also live in constant fear of becoming victims of crime in the drug or sex trafficking business. Immigrants work hard in the United States at physically demanding and low-wage jobs.

In conjunction with the first myth is the myth that immigrants cost taxpayers a lot. The fact is that they pay taxes but often do not reap the benefits of public assistance programs. Immigrants pay into Social Security but are not eligible to draw it. Additionally, immigrants serve in the military but cannot vote. The fact is that denying healthcare, even to undocumented immigrants, is more expensive for taxpayers (Ewing, 2003).

The third and fourth myths regard how often immigrants use the healthcare system and their lack of paying for healthcare. Many people believe that immigrants use the ED more than native-born citizens. The fact is that native-born citizens use healthcare significantly more than do immigrants because immigrants cannot afford healthcare. Using the ED occurs when medical conditions become life-threatening, not as a source of primary healthcare (Mohanty, 2012; Mohanty et al., 2005; Pandey & Kagotho, 2010). Furthermore, immigrants do not use healthcare because they cannot afford it. They pay taxes, which support public programs, but do not have access to them, and they often neglect their health because they cannot pay. In a study by Song et al. (2009) of Korean immigrants, the researchers found that those immigrants did not use healthcare precisely because they did not have money. However, those same people said that if they had insurance they would make use of healthcare services (Ewing, 2003; Mohanty, 2012).

Myth number five is that immigrants are unhealthy when they come to the United States. The fact is that they are healthy upon arrival to this country. However, generally after living in the United States for 5 years, their health worsens as a result of not receiving any healthcare (Mancuso, 2011; Pandey & Kagotho, 2010).

The last myth is one that relates to the attitudes of healthcare professionals. They believe that immigrants are not going to follow the instructions for treatment so why waste the time and money treating them. The fact is that many barriers exist which hinder immigrants from following healthcare instructions. Language, ethnic/cultural, financial, and travel barriers can prevent immigrants from being able to carry out health instructions (Luque, Raychowdhury, & Weaver, 2012; Mancuso, 2011; Squires & Anderson, 2015).

WHAT ARE THE RESULTS?

So, what are the results of denying healthcare to refugees and immigrants? Unfortunately, many U.S. citizens believe that denying care is less costly and cannot see the immediate and long-term implications for society. One effect is that children of refugees and immigrants do not receive immunizations or preventive care. Mothers are unable to initiate immunizations or to maintain the appropriate schedule, thus leading to outbreaks of diseases such as measles and chickenpox. One such example was in a California high school where a student of immigrant parents had tuberculosis that he spread to approximately one quarter of the other students.

Maternal/child health also suffers as the result of little to no prenatal healthcare. Preventable birth defects, such as those related to vitamin B deficiencies, abound. Additionally, poor maternal prenatal healthcare leads to low birth weight and generally unhealthy newborns. These babies often remain unhealthy in childhood and beyond, which leads to higher costs.

Adult healthcare is also impacted. Younger adult immigrants and refugees do not receive screening for infectious or chronic diseases or any healthcare education. For example, Museru et al. (2010) discussed the impact of immigrants who arrive in the United States with hepatitis B. They have limited access to healthcare and the disease progression can lead to serious complications and death. Furthermore, they carry a blood-borne chronic disease which could be transmitted to others and lead to a widespread outbreak. Older adults who already have chronic diseases are unable to manage these diseases adequately, thus leading to complications and comorbidities, which are more expensive to treat. End stage renal disease (ESRD) is one example. Undocumented immigrants with ESRD are unable to have dialysis on a regular basis or purchase essential medications. The result is that these individuals end up coming to the ED and require emergent dialysis. Again, this situation ultimately is more expensive than providing access to regular care (Ewing, 2003; Nandi, Loue, & Galea, 2009; Paylish, Noor, & Brandt, 2010).

BARRIERS TO HEALTHCARE ACCESS FOR IMMIGRANTS AND REFUGEES

A number of barriers prevent access to adequate and timely healthcare for immigrants and refugees, with the primary barrier being legislation. Individuals with immigrant/refugee status instead of citizenship are not eligible for public assistance. For those who are undocumented, fear of deportation hinders them from seeking healthcare unless the situation is life-threatening. Even for some legal immigrants, deportation remains a worry, and they are reluctant to seek healthcare.

Little or no healthcare coverage is a major barrier and deters immigrants from attending to their health needs unless absolutely critical. Although the prevailing thought among native-born U.S. citizens is that immigrants use the healthcare system much more often than them, the opposite is true. Immigrants and refugees pay out of pocket, and if they lack the finances, they do not seek healthcare. Often these individuals are employed at low-wage jobs that provide no health insurance or the cost of coverage in prohibitive.

Language and cultural barriers prevent initial contact with the healthcare system and/or follow-up care. U.S. healthcare professionals have proven to be less than sensitive to immigrants and refugees' cultural beliefs. Healthcare instructions are limited and usually need the services of an interpreter. In many healthcare facilities, families of patients are not allowed to interpret healthcare, so accessing someone who has medical interpreter training and is fluent in both languages can prove to be difficult. Furthermore, Western medicine does not acknowledge many cultural healthcare beliefs and dismiss them as foolish. The experiences of immigrants and refugees in the U.S. healthcare system can be quite frustrating and embarrassing to the point that patients choose not to return. Moreover, immigrants and refugees report an attitude of hostility from native-born U.S. citizens, including healthcare professionals, which only reinforces their reluctance to seek healthcare.

Many immigrants and refugees, especially women and the elderly, feel isolated even within their own communities. They may spend a significant part of the day alone while family members work. They lack a means of transportation, and thus, they are unable to travel to medical appointments. Additionally, this isolation may mean that many individuals lack awareness of community/neighborhood programs that are available (Hardy et al., 2012; Luque et al., 2012; Mancuso, 2011; Marrow, 2012; Nam, 2008; Pandey & Kagotho, 2010).

GAPS IN THE LITERATURE

One of the gaps in the literature noted by the author and stated by researchers is the diversity of immigrant population studied. A significant number of studies exist that have focused on Hispanic/Latino and Asian populations, but few have targeted African or Middle Eastern populations.

A second gap noted is the lack of studies of pregnant women and access to prenatal care. Although this population is especially vulnerable, a need exists to explore and understand more of the experiences of this population and how they might best be served.

The experience of healthcare professionals providing care to immigrants and refugees is a third gap noted. Some study reports noted statements and/or attitudes of healthcare professionals who provided a significant amount of care to immigrants. Healthcare professionals who chose to work with undocumented immigrants spoke of experiencing hostility from colleagues.

SUMMARY OF LITERATURE

In summary, the findings of the literature review demonstrate that immigrants and refugees have little or no access to healthcare or health-care coverage. Although they are relatively healthy upon arrival to the United States, their health worsens about 5 years after arrival because of major changes in their living and the lack of healthcare. Immigrants and refugees do not account for the majority of healthcare costs in the United States nor are they the most frequent users of EDs, rather native-born citizens are. Immigrants and refugees encounter multiple barriers in locating and accessing healthcare programs, and they are not looking for a hand out or to live off taxpayers' money. Without adequate healthcare, immigrants can create risks for public health as well as requiring more expensive emergent care for untreated chronic diseases.

POSSIBILITIES FOR RESOLUTION

Resolving the issues related to immigrant/refugee access to healthcare has not been an easy undertaking. One resolution noted in the literature review was to reverse the 5-year waiting period for immigrants and refugees to be eligible for healthcare funding. However, this reversal has not happened. Presently, after the 8-month assistance period is ended, immigrants and refugees are ineligible for Medicaid or Medicare Part A because they are Registered Provisional Immigrants (RPI). Being granted Lawfully Permanent Resident (LPR) status may take up to ten years, after which immigrants and refugees must wait another 5 years to be eligible for healthcare coverage under Medicaid or Medicare (Center for Medicare Advocacy, 2018). Under the current U.S. administration, changes to healthcare funding for refugees and immigrants are unlikely to take place.

The creation of racially, culturally, and ethnically sensitive local programs for immigrants, which provide health education and basic healthcare services, is another possibility. We also need to train bilingual individuals to help immigrants and refugees navigate the legal and healthcare systems in an efficient and timely manner. The Affordable Healthcare Act, often referred to as Obamacare, is also proving to help people in need of healthcare. The author is familiar with three clinics that provide healthcare to immigrants and refugees in her home state of Georgia. One is the Good News Clinic in Gainesville. The others are in Clarkston, home to the largest population of refugees and immigrants in the state. Those are the Georgia Refugee Health and Mental Health Clinic (GRHMHC) and the Grace Medical Village Clinic. Both of these clinics are staffed by volunteer healthcare providers and are funded by grants and donations.

REFERENCES

American College of Physicians. (2011). National immigration policy and access to health care. White paper. Retrieved from http://www.acponline.org/acp_policy/policies/natl_immigration_policy_access_healthcare_2011.pdf

Baiden, A. (2010). The impact of undocumented aliens on healthcare: The case of a Northern New Jersey Hospital. *Journal of Chi Eta Phi Sorority*, *54*(1), 5–6.

Burr, J., Gerst, K., Kwan, N., & Mutchler, J. (2009). Economic well-being and welfare program participation among older immigrants in the United States. *Generations, 32*(4), 53–60.

Center for Medicare Advocacy. (2018). Immigration reform and access to health care. Retrieved from http://www.medicareadvocacy.org

Centers for Medicare and Medicaid Services. (2018). Retrieved from https://www.cms.gov

Edberg, M., Cleary, S., & Vyas, A. (2011). A trajectory model for understanding and assessing health disparities in immigrant/refugee communities. *Journal of Immigrant and Minority Health, 13*(3), 576–584. doi:10.1007/s10903-010-9337-5

Ewing, W. (2003). *Not getting what they paid for: Limiting immigrants' access to benefits hurts families without reducing healthcare costs.* Washington, DC: Immigration Policy Center.

Ewing, W. (2012). Opportunity and exclusion: A brief history of U.S. immigration policy. Retrieved from http://immigrationpolicy.org/special-reports/opportunity-and-exclusion-brief-history-us-immigration-policy

Fix, M. & Passel, J. (1994). Immigration and immigrants: Setting the record straight. The Urban Institute website. Retrieved from http://webarchive.urban.org/publications/305184.html

Gusmano, M. (2012). Undocumented immigrants in the United States: U.S. health policy and access to care. The Hastings Center. Retrieved from http://www.undocumentedpatients.org/issuebrief/health-policy-and-access-to-care

Hardy, L., Getrich, C., Quezada, J., Guay, A., Michalowski, R., & Eric Henley, E. (2012). A call for further research on the impact of state-level immigration. *American Journal of Public Health, 102*(7), 1250–1254. doi:10.2105/AJPH.2011.300541

HealthCare.gov. (2013). The Patient Protection and Affordable Healthcare Act. Retrieved from http://www.healthcare.gov/law/full/index.html

Immigration Policy Center. (2013). Why don't they just get in line: The real story of getting a "green card" and coming to the United States legally. Retrieved from http://www.immigrationpolicy.org/just-facts/why-don%E2%80%99t-they-just-get-line

Luque, J., Raychowdhury, S., & Weaver, M. (2012). Health care provider challenges for reaching Hispanic immigrants with HPV vaccination in rural Georgia. *Rural and Remote Health, 12*(2), 1975.

Mancuso, L. (2011). Overcoming health literacy barriers: A model for action. *Journal of Cultural Diversity, 18*(2), 60–67.

Marrow, H. B. (2012). The power of local autonomy: Expanding health care to unauthorized immigrants in San Francisco. *Ethnic & Racial Studies, 35*(1), 72. doi:10.1080/01419870.2011.594168

Mohanty, S. (2012). Persistent disparities in cholesterol screening among immigrants to the United States. *International Journal for Equity in Health, 11*(1), 22–25. doi:10.1186/1475-9276-11-22

Mohanty, S., Woolhandler, S., Himmelstein, D., Pati, S., Carrasquillo, O., & Bor, D. (2005). Health care expenditures of immigrants in the United States: A nationally representative analysis. *American Journal of Public Health, 95*(8), 1431–1438. doi:10.2105/AJPH.2004.044602

Museru, O., Vargas, M., Kinyua, M., Alexander, K., Franco-Paredes, C., & Oladele, A. (2010). Hepatitis B virus infection among refugees resettled in the U.S.: High prevalence and challenges in access to health care. *Journal of Immigrant and Minority Health, 12*(6), 823–827. doi:10.1007/s10903-010-9335-7

Nam, Y. (2008). Welfare reform and older immigrants' health insurance coverage. *American Journal of Public Health, 98*(11), 2029–2034. doi:10.2105/AJPH.2007.120675

Nandi, A., Loue, S., & Galea, S. (2009). Expanding the universe of universal coverage: The population health argument for increasing coverage for immigrants. *Journal of Immigrant Minority Health, 11*(6), 433–436. doi:10.1007/s10903-009-9267-2

Pandey, S., & Kagotho, N. (2010). Health insurance disparities among immigrants: Are some legal immigrants more vulnerable than others? *Health and Social Work, 35*(4), 267–279. doi:10.1093/hsw/35.4.267

Paylish, C., Noor, S., & Brandt, J. (2010). Somali immigrant women and the American health care system: Discordant beliefs, divergent expectations, and silent worries. *Social Science and Medicine, 71*(2), 353–361. doi:10.1016/j.socscimed.2010.04.010

Refugee Health Technical Assistance Center. (2011). Retrieved from http://refugeehealthta.org/access-to-care

Song, H., Han, H., Lee, J., Kim, J., Kim, K., Ryu, J., & Kim, M. (2010). Does access to care still affect health care utilization by immigrants? Testing of an empirical explanatory model of health care utilization by Korean American immigrants with high blood pressure. *Journal of Immigrant and Minority Health, 12*(4), 513–519. doi:10.1007/s10903-009-9276-1

Squires, D., & Anderson, C. (2015). U.S. Health care from a global perspective: Spending, use of services, prices, and health in

13 countries. Retrieved from The Commonwealth Fund website: http://www.commonwealthfund.org

State of Georgia Refugee Health Guideline Manual. (n.d.). Retrieved from https://dph.georgia.gov/sites/dph.georgia.gov/files/RHP-Refugee%20Health%20Guideline%20Manual_1.pdf

Tavis, A. (2010). Healthcare for all: Ensuring states comply with the equal protection rights of legal immigrants. *Boston College Law Review, 51*(5), 1627–1668. Retrieved from http://lawdigitalcommons.bc.edu/bclr/vol51/iss5/7

Viladrich, A. (2012). Beyond welfare reform: Reframing undocumented immigrants' entitlement to health care in the United States, a critical review. *Social Science and Medicine, 74*(6), 822–829. doi:10.1016/j.socscimed.2011.05.050

From International Physician to U.S. Nurse Practitioner: Multiple Life History Study

Krisola Marcano
Charlotte Ndema
Nancy Martinez
Jennifer Azelton

This study presents life histories of two international physicians in the United States transitioning to nurse practitioners (NPs) enrolled in an international physician to NP bridge program at Kennesaw State University (KSU). A nursing shortage exists in the United States, and the American Association of Colleges of Nursing suggested reaching out beyond the usual recent high school graduate pool to target underrepresented and nontraditional groups to fill the shortage (Grossman & Jorda, 2008). Specifically, the National Institute for Health Care Management called for an increase in NPs as insurance coverage on Americans expands with the Affordable Care Act and the U.S. populace grows with an aging baby boomer population (Iglehart, 2014). The pool of foreign-educated physicians (FEPs) is also expanding, but numerous FEPs work for low-pay jobs or they are unemployed (Flowers & Olenick, 2014; Grossman & Jorda, 2008). The FEP pool is ethnically and culturally diverse. This diversity would help to increase the number of minority nurses and provide healthcare to the increasingly diverse U.S. population. Also, most of the FEPs are men, and they could increase the male nurses' population in the United States (Grossman & Jorda, 2008).

According to the American Medical Association, 23% of the U.S. physician population is international medical graduates (Grossman & Jorda, 2008). Obtaining certification to practice in the United States, however, requires strenuous application. FEPs must pass their United States Medical Licensing Examination (USMLE), become Educational Commission for Foreign Medical Graduates (ECFMG) certified, then apply to residency programs, and, if they are lucky, considered for a competitive interview out of hundreds of qualified candidates trying to fill one spot (Pande, 2014; Peterson, Pandya, & Leblang, 2014). Pande (2014) examined the international mobility of physicians by paralleling the laws that regulate the practice of foreign-trained physicians in the United States and eight other countries: India, China, the Philippines, Germany, the United Kingdom, Denmark, Australia, and Israel. There are two laws that regulate the practice of medicine in the United States: the General Agreement on Trade in Services (GATS) and the North American Free Trade Agreement (NAFTA; Pande, 2014). The GATS is the major agreement that could theoretically impact the movement of physicians but seems to have had limited effect on their migration (Pande, 2014). Trading conditions have become more restrictive through NAFTA, which enables Canadian and Mexican physicians to work in the United States above workers from other countries (Pande, 2014).

International medical graduates from other countries must meet the same requirements as U.S.-trained physicians, no matter their country of origin. In 2002, according to the National Resident Matching Program, 6,585 FEPs applied to residency that year; 3,427 or 52% were offered positions, whereas of the 16,661 U.S. medical graduate active applicants that year, 14,876 or 89.3% were offered a position (Pande, 2014). Many of the foreign physicians were not considered and remained unemployed or settled for low-wage jobs, even in hospital settings (Grossman & Jorda, 2008; Hafer, 2011). The unemployment or underemployment of this skilled foreign workforce touched the hearts of leaders from two federally funded nursing institutions to create programs to re-educate FEPs to NPs. Florida International University School of Nursing and Kennesaw State University WellStar School of Nursing have been the only schools to embrace the challenge (Grossman & Jorda, 2008; Hafer, 2011).

WellStar College of Health and Human Services' associate dean, Dr. David Bennett, was moved to do something after witnessing many foreign-trained physicians serve as translators in their community clinics because they could not practice (Hafer, 2011). Many of these physicians had passed all of their qualifying exams for a U.S. medical license and spent thousands of dollars on review courses but were unable to enter a residency program due to unfavorable selection policies in which new graduate medical students received top preference (Hafer, 2011). Dr. Bennett's compassionate heart led to the creation of the WellStar BSN-MSN Family Nurse Practitioner Program for Foreign Physicians (Hafer, 2011).

TRANSITION THEORY

Transition theory supports the idea of FEP transition to NP. According to Goodman, Schlossberg, and Anderson (2006), a transition is "any event or non-event that results in changed relationships, routines, assumptions, and roles" (p. 53). Individuals face different kinds of change over their lifespan, which are triggered by natural events of human evolution. The life histories of these foreign physicians who come to the United States show several adjustments including, but not limited to, immigration, linguistic barriers, environment, and major professional adaptations. They had to go through a transition process in order to fit in.

According to Meleis (2010), transition theory is integrative and acts upon individuals who are experimenting in a change process and who likely show more vulnerability. Foreign physicians in this study were the people experiencing a transitional process while trying to earn a living in the United States. Meleis goes on to describe the transition process as a framework made of three important steps: the nature of the transition with concepts including types, patterns, and properties; the transition conditions with concepts including facilitators and inhibitors, both personal and community; and the patterns of response including outcome indicators. Meleis's transition theory applied to the FEP and covered their course of change from foreign physician to U.S. NP. These physicians experienced a professional paradigm shift from being a doctor in their respective homeland to becoming a nurse in the United States. As foreign doctors, they also encountered many challenges such as environmental and cultural change, language barriers, professional limitation, and immigration issues. In accordance with Meleis's three-step process theory, first, the FEP's nature of transition involved shifting from doctor to nurse; second, the transition conditions included acceptance into a college degree bridge program; and third, a pattern of response to the transition which exhibited struggling versus successful graduation and ease into society as an NP.

SIGNIFICANCE

This study documents the experiences of the participants in an innovative and unique way. The study also shed light on medical training and healthcare outside the United States, revealing cultural differences that may affect future training of FEPs and further develop the multicultural communities they work in. The need for NPs continues to grow, and providing research on FEPs strengthens the argument for such a program to relieve the nursing shortage.

THE LITERATURE

Research on foreign physicians transitioning to NPs is scarce and reiterates the need for further study. This review focuses on all studies specific to foreign physician migration and highlights common themes through several qualitative papers. Furthermore, it assesses research on U.S. needs for patient care providers, migrant location choices, role transition from physician to nurse, and suggestion of areas needing more study.

In assessing the need versus overpopulation of patient care providers, Libby, Zhou, and Kindig (1997) created and tested a model to predict U.S. physician requirements for the future. They determined that minority providers were more likely to practice in areas with large minority populations; so in order to meet the growing minority populations by year 2010, Hispanic and black physicians would need to double and white physicians shrink by two fifths (Libby et al., 1997). These numbers would then need to continue at such a rate for racial and ethnic disparities to level out by 2060. The authors suggest increasing the number of foreign physician immigrants to help meet goals more efficiently and benefit immigrant minority populations within the United States (Libby et al., 1997).

Many immigrants move in order to access better pay and quality of life, and they often travel from low-resource countries (Chen et al., 2010; Vapor & Xu, 2011). In comparison, a large European study assessing healthcare worker migration discovered that labor market restrictions, improvement of salaries, and working conditions within the home countries were improving and such acted as a barrier to movement (Ognyanova, Maier, Wismar, Girasek, & Busse, 2012).

The immense and ever-changing private insurance system within the United States is also mentioned as a challenging area during emigration and transition (Chen et al., 2010). Policies around the world regarding pay for healthcare vary greatly from financially driven healthcare systems to government driven and even barter driven in low-resource countries (Hamric, Hanson, Tracy, & O'Grady, 2014). Learning the U.S. system takes time, and fear of litigation limits practice among many FEPs who are scared of being sued for incorrect practice (Chen et al., 2010; Jauregui & Xu, 2010).

Many barriers have been described, but positive themes include greater financial gain, empathy toward minority patients, and experience with diseases uncommon in the United States (Chen et al., 2010). It should be noted that FEPs bring unique skills, including broad knowledge of diseases rare to Western medicine, such as meningitis and tuberculosis, plus a greater sense of empathy toward minority patients (Chen et al., 2010).

Finding research specific to FEPs transitioning to U.S. NPs presented a challenge due to limited literature, but all reports documented successful transitions and encouraged further investigation. A common theme among FEPs who became NPs was their difficulty in becoming certified as physicians in the United States due to the expenses involved in passing the USMLE and slim opportunities for attaining residency placement (Pande, 2014; Peterson et al., 2014). As a result, many FEPs worked in low-paying, unsatisfying jobs such as medical assistants (Flowers & Olenick, 2014). Grossman and Jorda (2008) performed an investigation focused on the new American in nursing accelerated program at the Nicole Wertheim College of Nursing and Health Sciences at Florida International University. The program was directed to FEPs who were U.S. residents, unemployed or underemployed, and desired to obtain a bachelor's degree in nursing in the Unites States. The researchers described characteristics of the immigrants in nursing accelerated programs, including prerequisites, durability, awareness of credits for general education, and matriculation of nursing courses (Grossman & Jorda, 2008). In addition, the authors explored outcomes of the program such as level of socialization, degree of critical thinking skills, and pass rates for National Council Licensure Exam for Registered Nurses (NCLEX-RN®) exhibited by FEPs in comparison to generic baccalaureate nursing students (Grossman & Jorda, 2008). Results demonstrated that FEPs had higher than average NCLEX-RN pass rates plus carried significantly strong clinical and critical thinking skills but struggled in adjusting "philosophy based on care instead of cure" (Grossman & Jorda, 2008, p. 549). Also, the research mentions the value of such a program as an option to improve the nursing shortage with the added benefit of a needed cultural diversity within the field (Grossman & Jorda, 2008).

Research completed by Garrido, Simon, Purnell, Scisney-Matlock, and Pontious (2016) describes andragogies and technology-based teaching methods currently used to increase cultural competence for adult students who were FEPs in an American BSN-MSN bridge program at Florida International University. The study involved a comparison of students in their first versus final semester and assessed cultural competence and language improvement over the course of the program (Garrido et al., 2016).

Culturally competent care improved among students through the use of simulation and online education methods (Garrido et al., 2016). These methods included cultural case simulations through a manikin with two-way microphone between student and teacher, online discussions, and several writing assignments on providing culturally competent care as providers (Garrido et al., 2016). In an additional finding, it was assessed that written English proved a great difficulty for a significant number of these students, but all felt that they had improved and appreciated the opportunity for progression through the use of faculty and the university writing center (Garrido et al., 2016). This chapter exemplifies the need for schools to offer assistance to FEPs through the use of a writing center and hands-on learning in order for the students to develop a better understanding of culture and language communication.

Alpert, Yucha, and Atienza (2013) explored a qualitative perspective of an accelerated family nurse practitioner (FNP) program offered to foreign medical doctors who also earned a BSN. Researchers found that for economic reasons many Filipino physicians returned to school to become nurses in order to immigrate to the United States with the hope of a better quality of life (Alpert et al., 2013). The academic program was a master's degree course at the University of Nevada, Las Vegas, with the collaboration of Saint Jude College in the Philippines, and it graduated 76 students between 2006 and 2010, with all pupils passing the national certification FNP exam during the first attempt (Alpert et al., 2013).

A phenomenological study by Vapor and Xu (2011) collected experiences of FEPs from the Philippines who became nurses in the United States and discovered several struggles in transitioning roles. The first theme was of embarrassment at the thought of a demotion from doctor to nurse plus fear of greater expectations in work performance due to true level of education (Vapor & Xu, 2011). A second theme was that FEPs believed they would experience financial gain but in reality, though the salary was greater in the United States, quality of life was not improved, and according to partici-pants, in the Philippines, doctors only make $300 to $1,000 per month but live a grandiose life with butlers and maids (Vapor & Xu, 2011). The third and final theme disclosed unhappiness among FEPs due to labor-intensive demands as bedside nurses (Vapor & Xu, 2011). At the end of the study, it should be noted that half of the respondents decided to pursue degrees as advanced practice nurses, including NPs, as a solution for more autonomy, better pay, and use of their medical expertise (Vapor & Xu, 2011).

Jauregui and Xu (2010) did a phenomenological study examining transitional issues faced by FEPs from the Philippines who became NPs in the United States. The greatest challenges noted were navigation of the U.S. health system and insurance regulations, reduced scope of practice in comparison to when they were medical doctors, and fearfulness of lawsuits (Jauregui & Xu, 2010). On the other hand, they felt great occupational fulfilment as NPs compared to staff nurses and their medical schooling and experience eased the switch (Jauregui & Xu, 2010).

The few studies available seem to boost the need for more research on the transition from FEP to NP. It has been documented that FEPs transitioning to NPs feel greater job satisfaction versus those that work lower education medical jobs in the United States (Flowers & Olenick, 2014; Jauregui & Xu, 2010). Further study of motivational factors for migration and FEP transition to NP with discussion of barriers and suggestions on overcoming challenges, such as language, cultural, practical, and ethical customs, may provide support for future FEPs, NPs, healthcare systems, and educational programs.

METHODOLOGY

DESIGN

The design was a multiple life history that included narrative analysis of participants' information. Participants provided a descriptive narration of their experience becoming international medical doctors and transitioning to NPs in the United States.

SAMPLE

Two international medical doctors comprise the study sample for this research project.

They were both over 18 years of age and attended the foreign physician MSN-FNP program. The protection of rights of the subject sample was through the use of pseudonymous names to identify each participant during the research. The study was approved by the university Institutional Review Board (IRB).

SETTING

The setting to collect the research data was at Kennesaw State University (KSU) in a secluded study room within the nursing building. This place provided a convenient and proper environment to promote attention and observation throughout the interview with a low grade of interruption, and also with an adequate level of comfort and privacy for the participant and interviewer.

INSTRUMENTATION

The instrument for gathering data in this project was the interviewer, who used a semi-structured interview guide. Each interview was audio-recorded and transcribed. The data were content analyzed, and a list of themes was generated.

The semi-structured interview guide:

1. Tell me about yourself and where you grew up.

2. What influenced your decision to become a doctor?

3. Describe your medical school experience and certification process.

4. What factors led to your emigration?

5. Why did you choose to transition from an MD to NP?

6. What have been your biggest challenges through this transition?

7. How did you overcome said challenges?

8. Who or what have been your sources of support?

9. What is your goal as an NP?

RIGOR

The study depends on reports of the participants' experiences from childhood through adulthood. Discussion among the research team members ensured consistent interpretation of results, which was validated with the participants.

RESULTS

The participants interviewed were two female international physicians who came to live in the United States for different reasons, one political and one for family. They experienced many changes through immigration, environmental, sociocultural, and professional transitions in order to create new conditions of life in the United States. This study focuses on the professional shift undergone by both participants. The foreign physicians were chosen for their personal life experience in becoming FNPs in the United States.

CHRISTY'S INTERVIEW RESULTS

Persecution

According to Levine (2001), persecution can take on many forms and may include torture, beatings, psychological/sexual abuse, deprivation, and burns. Persecution in her primary country was what led Christy to flee her country and start her life and medical career elsewhere. She stated that the dictator, who was in charge at the time, influenced the poor population into persecuting those whom had education. This education was equated to wealth and privilege and was, therefore, to be hated by those who had less or who were not educated. She saw her colleagues being harassed by her very own employers, and sometimes they would turn up dead. Other times, there would be random drive-by shootings on police officers while they were eating at a coffee shop. With the lurking danger in her life and jeopardy just by doing her job, it became necessary to seek an asylum in another country to be able to work and live her life in safety.

> In my country, education was free to everyone. Anyone who wanted an education could get one without having to pay for it. The government paid for the education. Seventeen years ago a dictator who was in power, accused us of being capitalized and rich which wasn't true. I was a regular citizen in my country and I chose to go to school. This dictator divided the country. He was a military dictator who convinced the poor people that the doctors, lawyers, and educated people were bad. He manipulated the country and won the elections. Educated people were being killed for nothing.

I had a college and ex-classmate-physician who was murdered by criminals without reason. Cases like this occurred every day without justice or investigation. People were kidnapped and killed. If they did not have money to pay for the return of a kidnapped person, they were killed; it was crazy!

Sanctuary

Christy had to seek sanctuary somewhere after suffering the persecution and turmoil that was going on in her native country. The need for sanctuary was a strong feeling and desire in Christy to have somewhere safe to live and work without fear of death or persecution. It was a life or death decision to seek sanctuary somewhere else. She left her country and worked in Germany because she had a valid medical doctor's degree in Europe. While abroad, transition was easier because her native language was the same but she still did not feel safe. Eventually, she decided to come to the United States where she had great opportunities to make the country her new home. Even though it implied a new start with a new language, a new profession, and different culture, she expressed gratitude that she could walk the streets at night or leave her window blinds up without the fear of being shot at.

> I left my country looking for a safe place to live. My first option was a country in Europe, because I had a valid surgical medical doctor degree. Medical degrees are accepted and valid in European countries. It was easier in this country because people spoke my language; therefore, it was an easy decision. After I was working as a doctor in that country and interacting with the people, I did not feel safe. I decided to come to America which became my new safe home. There were a lot of wonderful opportunities for people who wanted to give the best of their effort.

Discovery

After finding her new home in the United States, Christy discovered that she needed to find a way to be able to practice medicine in the United States. What Christy discovered was her new future and life in her new home. She had to make a choice of whether to pursue a medical degree in the United States, since her physician license from her native country was not recognized in the United States, or choose another path in the healthcare field. If she chose to pursue her medical doctorate degree, it would mean repeating residency after passing her medical boards. This would have equated to several years or more before she could practice medicine again. Christy, however, discovered that she could become a useful healthcare professional through the NP program for international physicians at KSU. This was the perfect avenue for her to be able to practice medicine again in the same way she practiced in her native country, a place where medical doctors are more like American nurses. She discovered that she could make a new life for herself in the United States and still practice medicine, just in a different role than she experienced in her native country.

> Since I decided to come to the United States, I studied English as my first goal. I had a friend who told me about this University and the Nurse Practitioner Master's Program for International Physicians. He told me that this program could give me the opportunity to be a healthcare provider in the U.S., but I did not know what it meant, nor what a nurse practitioner was. I did not have any idea about my current profession; it was a major discovery. I tried to become a medical doctor in the U.S., but it was almost impossible for many factors. I figured that I would be the best nurse practitioner in the U.S. or be a surgical medical doctor nowhere. When I got the letter of acceptance from KSU that I got in, it opened the door to all of the possibilities in this country.

Challenge/Language Barrier

For Christy, the language barrier presented a formidable challenge. Not being able to communicate to those around her in her new safe homeland was very distressing to her. This handicap kept her from being able to fully integrate and participate in her new home. During Christy's interview, the presence of a language barrier was noted as a challenge in her process of becoming an FNP in the United States. Christy stated that she had a very remedial knowledge of English before coming to the United States and realized that English preparation was very important for her entry into the American healthcare field. Christy noted that she spent 3 years studying English in order to qualify for application at KSU. In addition, she expressed desire to continue her language education.

> I did not study English before because it was not necessary in my country. I just had the basic knowledge of it. I did not speak English when I came to the U.S. It was very frustrating because I could not understand when people talked to me. I started to learn English

as my second language. It took me about three years of hard and persistent work, and attendance to several institutions such as the Interactive Technical College, Georgia State University, and Chattahoochee Technical College. I went through all of this effort because I decided I wanted to be able to practice in the healthcare field in my new country. I have been speaking English for six years now, but I know that I must keep learning, therefore I am planning on a second major in English at the University.

Perseverance

A highlight from Christy's interview was her personal and career perseverance. Since Christy's adolescence and young adult years, she was very clear about her desire to study and serve in the healthcare field, a trait which was encouraged by her mother. In Christy's country, as the same in the United States, medical school student application, master of public health, and graduate ophthalmology specialty selection have a strict and competitive process. Christy showed great success in her schoolwork and had consistent evaluation and supervision by highly qualified medical staff as an undergrad, graduate doctoral student, internal medicine intern, general surgery resident, master of public health, and ophthalmology specialty practice.

After completing the highest education level as a medical doctor, several political and safety issues in Christy's country influenced her decision to immigrate to a safer place. This implicated a new start to several aspects of Christy's life including language, profession, and finances, all with very little social support. Despite the lack of support, Christy always persevered and continued in her pursuit to serve as a healthcare provider and active community member. She discovered a different and special path, which coordinated with the way she was prepared as a medical doctor in her native country and offered her an opportunity as a highly qualified health professional in her new country.

> Always, I have been a very active, enthusiastic, optimistic, and proactive person. I think that the biggest feature of my personality is perseverance and a strong sense of belief in a better future. My mother was always with me motivating me to follow my heart and inspiration to work for the people. My medical school time was eight years after I graduated from high school. I was in a select group of people trying to go into medical school. There were about eight hundred applications to trying to go in and only five hundred were accepted, and I was one of them. I graduated as a surgeon medical doctor. Then, I did

two years of internship on the four main specialties such as internal medicine, general surgery, GYN/OB, and pediatric. Then, I did two years of residency of general surgery. Also, I did a master of public health. Finally, I did the ophthalmology specialty which was three years after a very strict and competitive process of selection, which just accepted seven physicians of more than three hundred applications, and I was one of them. Since I came to the U.S., I had the desire to practice in the healthcare field which motivated me to consider other wonderful and alternative options. Because I am a healthcare provider in my heart, I did not need a doctor degree to help people to keep their health. I just wanted be a proactive and useful member of my new community. Becoming a medical doctor in the U.S. is almost impossible for international physicians because the cost, the bureaucracy, the time, few residency places, many limitations, and no specialty accreditation. It implicated a start over of everything.

Hope/Faith

As a new immigrant, Christy expressed deep hope and faith that her future in the United States could be safer and better than the country she came from. During Christy's interview, she transmitted that even though she confronted many obstacles and experienced a difficult move, she was still positive, hopeful, and faithful toward her future in the United States. In addition, Christy stated her hopefulness that the NP program for international physicians at KSU will open its doors again for other medical doctors like her.

When I came to this country, I knew that something good would happen with my life, I felt safe and I knew that God would help me to find the real path of my vocation of services. Sometimes I felt scared because many obstacles and difficulties were there, but my faith maintained me up, waiting for the great opportunity . . . and it became a reality when I was accepted at nurse practitioner program master for international physicians.

Gratitude

By the end of the interview, Christy stated phrases of gratitude toward God and life because the nursing program offered her a dream opportunity to become a healthcare provider in the form of an FNP. She explained that the NP program for international physicians was convenient and well-suited to her for circumstances and reasons that she did not understand but she expressed appreciation for the positive impact of this program on her life. In addition, Christy showed pride in her choice to become an FNP and manifested satisfaction and happiness in following her passion of service within the healthcare field. At the same time, Christy stated that she was very proud of other international physicians choosing to become FNPs in the United States because the nation has a huge need for those professionals in the workforce.

> I need to express my deep gratefulness to God, life, and the nursing school for giving me the opportunity of my life which changed my destiny ... I think that thank you is not enough to express my happiness and grateful feeling for them!

EMMA'S INTERVIEW RESULTS

Frustration

Emma encountered tremendous frustration during her transition from MD to FNP. Her frustrations were evident in numerous circumstances and expressed as a feeling of hindrance in achieving her personal goals and powerlessness to change the situation. The lack of residency training in her country took her to a foreign land to pursue further studies. Despite obtaining that specialization, she had to move to the United States against her will for family reasons. She had never been to the United States before, and she knew nothing about this new country. She resisted the change and went through difficult moments. She kept on looking behind wanting to go back to what she knew and what was familiar to her. Learning a new language was a frustration and common theme throughout her journey, and once settled in the United States, she encountered a major professional challenge in the initial transition to a registered nurse. She felt belittled at times and vulnerable during that period.

> They did not have residency training in my country at that time. You had to go out of the country for specialization back then. I had no idea what the U.S. looked like. I never wanted to move to the U.S. I truly did not want to. When I came to the U.S., the transition was not easy for me. I was down casted. I always looked back at what I left behind. Not practicing in the U.S. as a medical doctor was

truly depressing for me. I wanted to take my 2 younger children back to France to live. I was in the states for about 6–7 years before sitting down for the medical exam boards. I was learning English, that's a lot! Some of the challenges were not truly welcome because they would dig the hole more under our feet, you know like, there were some challenges where some colleagues would make things so hard and make me look like a dummy . . . why am I being belittled. I think I was really vulnerable, I was not strong. So my challenge from MD to nurse, not nurse practitioner but RN was that I was so vulnerable during that period. It was very difficult, I guess at my age to get jobs.

Lost

Emma conveyed that she felt lost, off track, and unable to find her way during and after her move to the United States. English was not her first language and she did not speak fluently or understand English well. This created an initial, literal sense of being lost, unable to communicate her basic needs to other people. Emma had never visited the United States before and knew very little. She never wanted to move to the United States. Her husband on the other hand loved the United States, spoke English as his first language, and was integrated while Emma felt lost. She finally took all the requested medical boards to practice in the United States after about 14 years. She even got five residency interviews but could not secure a position because she was not well adapted to the system.

I am from the French speaking part of Cameroon and my husband is from the English speaking one. Only French is spoken in France so our children spoke only French. My husband wanted his children to speak English. As we were having our children in a French speaking country, it was imperative for him to have his children speak English. Also, he loved the U.S., visited many times. I knew nothing about the U.S. My husband moved to U.S. as he felt in love with the U.S. My husband only came to the U.S.; many times before. Not the rest of the family. I had no idea what the U.S. looked like. I never wanted to move to the U.S. I truly did not want to. I was lost wondering what I was doing in a strange land. At that point, I realized I needed to be there for my kids. I got 5 interviews but could not secure a residency spot. I was back to my baseline. I am ECFMG certified in U.S. officially an MD with no residency training; now what? I asked myself.

Language Barrier

A frequent theme for Emma that molded with other concepts was the language barrier she faced. This figurative wall prevented her from communicating appropriately and limited her cultural understanding plus personal needs, access to jobs, and academic progression. Emma spoke French from her native land. She had to learn how to write in English and understand academic English, all while struggling with the spoken word. The language barrier, although reduced as an FNP student, was still a difficult reality for her at times.

> When you saw "nurse practitioner" you were thinking "nurse" all the time? That was one of the reasons why I didn't want to come to the U.S. because I wasn't speaking English. Coming from my country, I am French-speaking and my English was very rudimentary. The English I learned back home was British English so I was lost each time someone else was talking. It was horrible.

Hope

Emma displayed hope several times in the interview. This was demonstrated as an expressed sentiment of positive expectation for the future and ability to overcome her initial frustrations. Her husband knew that his children would have more opportunities if they grew up in the United States, and Emma showed commitment to his decision. During her time of difficulty applying for a medical residency program, she was offered an interview for the FNP program for foreign physicians at KSU. It was during this meeting that her hope was ignited by Dr. King who shed light on what the FNP role was. She successfully went through the accelerated BSN program and felt thrilled to go through the MSN education. She was looking forward to her graduation day because becoming a primary care provider in the United States was her ultimate goal.

> [My husband] wanted a safe life and a better educational system for his children like any good father. I had no idea about what the program was about exactly before my interview. I was wondering what a family nurse practitioner role was. I hesitated going for the interview. I was encouraged by my family and friends to make the move. At the end of the interview, Dr. King explained to me how a family nurse practitioner works.

> She told me FNP can work independently under very light phy-
> sician's control. She made it clear to me I can work independently
> after I graduate as a FNP and not like a bedside nurse. I was like
> really? After the nurse school ended and I started nurse practitioner
> program that adversity became instantly a plus to me. I'm actually
> excited, I'm loving it. For me, to tell you the truth, I'm looking
> forward and I can't wait to graduate now that I have seen a nurse
> practitioner working.

Joy

Toward the end of the interview, Emma voiced great joy with her current
state, a feeling of triumph and rejoicing to God for her success despite
the tribulations. She specifically identified that she had no remorse at
becoming an FNP and was delighted in the opportunity given to her by
KSU. Her English skills had also tremendously improved and in a breach
of the language barrier, she felt she could go even further in her studies
if she was a younger age.

> I like what I am doing and looking forward to become a NP. I
> have no regret. I bless God for Kennesaw because if I was a little
> bit younger I could do a PhD in English because of my passage,
> my transition to Kennesaw. They push me to write, write, write!
> I'm like, these people are killing me with writing, but it's a bless-
> ing. When I look at my writing that I took to the writing center
> now versus three years ago, they are like, "Oh my gosh! You have
> tremendously improved."

Caring

Emma understood how important the principle of caring was to nursing.
She expressed a desire to give back to the less privileged in a holistic way,
not only focusing on their disease but also acting as an advocate for her
patients. To further exemplify her caring role, Emma wanted to give back
to the community. She came from a modest background and through her
own transition understood what it felt like to be in need and was ready
to serve wherever she was sent.

> I want to serve the community. That would be my calling, underserved
> populations in the community. I just want to serve the underserved. I don't

care if they are English-speaking, French-speaking, or Japanese-speaking. One word, underserved. I am from a very modest background, that's the reason I'm happy, I'm content. I want to serve the underserved in the U.S., outside of the U.S., wherever I'll be sent, I'll do it God willing.

Intelligence

Emma's extensive resume displays her intelligence, her natural ability to learn and retain knowledge. Emma had to take a very competitive exam to get into medical school in her country, and then after practicing as a general practitioner she moved to Europe to complete a fellowship specialization. She practiced as a surgeon then moved to the United States with her family where she passed all the medical doctor licensing boards, completed a master of public health, and now plans to graduate with an additional master of science in nursing. This incredible display of intelligence shows the wealth of talent possessed by Emma.

> To enter in medical school back then, you needed to be really smart. I was very smart. All candidates for medical school needed to take a competitive exam in which 42 students were chosen among 6 to 9 thousand candidates nationwide. I went to [Europe], and did specialize … for 4 years. Then I worked for 6 years between as a surgeon. I passed all my board exams and was certified as a physician to practice medicine in the U.S., went to do a Master degree in Public Health for 2 years. I got my MPH in the U.S.

Strong Support System

Throughout the time of struggle after immigration, Emma expressed frustration and faced defeat but stayed steady in her pursuits through the strong support system of her family and friends. This group of people constantly and unwaveringly encouraged and reinforced her goals through their support. Emma's family, including her husband, sister, and children, plus close friends, demonstrated a loving and loyal bond to her. They were her support system and stood by her all the way through. They prayed for her and with her. They were her comfort and listening ear when she wanted to vent about her problems, and the shoulder on which she sometimes cried.

> I wanted to just drop everything and go but I have a good support system and family too. My husband first and I have some true friends

who I call and turn to many times when I wanted to quit during the nurse/RN study. My sister just said, stick in there, try your best, this is an open door. You know there will always be challenges. Family, friends and husband, and my children. I have 4 grown children.

Finances

Emma went through many resources to find good schools for her children and self. Above all, she was well informed on how and where to find school loans. Emma voiced gratitude for the advanced U.S. educational system that permitted her and her children to take loans in pursuit of higher education and a better quality of life.

> Well in my country of origin, we don't have big loans to become a physician but here we do; I know because one of my daughters, she's a doctor now. She's doing her residency. That's one of the things that keeps me going, I can see the loans we had to take! A lot of money! It is like a mortgage. God bless America for this opportunity [to take loans].

DISCUSSION

This study identified several concepts during the evaluation of results of the interviews, which were noted on individuals in a transitional process. According to Meleis (2010), transistion theory is an integrative theory that acts upon individuals who are experiencing changes. These changes require an individual to adapt to a new situation or environment according to life circumstances, and which is communicated as the individual's ability to cope. Transition theory involves five essential properties: awareness, engagement, change and difference, time span, and critical points and events (Meleis, Sawyer, Im, Hilfinger-Messias, & Schumacher, 2000).

The investigators identified four common concepts from this qualitative research, which showed that two individuals with different histories could go through a transition process and develop the ability to cope in their new environment and situations. During Christy's and Emma's interviews, these four concepts were hope, discovery, challenge, and gratefulness.

The first common concept identified was hope. Christy's hope was noted throughout the interview. Since she started to talk, she emphasized her wish to have a regular life in a safe place, which could bring a better opportunity to live and develop her potential as a healthcare professional. She confronted many limitations, barriers, and difficulties, but all of these obstacles made Christy develop a deep and strong sense of hope for a better future. Emma initially expressed a hope for the betterment of her children, similar to Christy's hope for her mother to live a life of security in a new society. They also shared a common desire to become proficient healthcare providers after struggling to achieve the status of medical doctor through the rigorous U.S. qualification system. At the end of each interview, a conveyed sense of hope for their futures in the United States as working NPs was shown as the ultimate desire and now within grasp. They then concluded with a hopefulness for other international physicians who come to the United States searching for a better future that they may find the same or similar opportunities offered to them.

The second common concept identified was discovery. When Christy came to the United States, she was constantly discovering. From Christy's start, she did not know what to do for work in the new country because her medical doctor preparation was not accredited. In a hopeful effort, she discovered several opportunities to advance her career. In chronological order, she discovered English preparation was needed to join the U.S. workforce and she found language classes. She then discovered that work with children as a nanny was an immediate solution to her labor and financial situation. Next, she learned that the healthcare field in the United States was vast and offered other options for international physicians, with the final discovery of the Family Nurse Practitioner program for FEPs at KSU. Emma's timeline of discovery in the United States started the same as Christy's with the search and finding of an English language class. She then went on and utilized her newfound communication skills to pursue further education with the completion of a Master of Public Health and a concordant job with the U.S. Veterans Affairs in order to work and make money. Then, just like Christy, she was invited to interview for the FNP bridge program at KSU, where she discovered the role of an NP and successfully began her entry into the U.S. health system as a healthcare provider.

The third core concept identified was challenge, and Christy's life had always been filled with challenges, starting with when she was a young adult applying to, then completing medical school in her hometown. When Christy immigrated to the United States, she discovered sanctuary and faced challenges at the same time, in order to adapt herself to a new environment and culture.

Christy described her education at KSU's nursing school as the most challenging goal. Learning a new profession, in a foreign language, in a different country was very difficult. She believed that she proved her strength in overcoming these challenges through persistence in meeting the ultimate goal of becoming an NP. Emma academically went through the same challenges as Christy with acceptance to and graduation from a doctorate degree program followed by specialization in a precise area of medicine. The specific challenges of learning a new language and culture resonated in both Emma's and Christy's interviews. Although both women were proficient in medicine, the difficulty of relearning everything and becoming capable enough to explain and educate patients on a provider level was especially tough. Emma, like Christy, was able to conquer these challenges through completion of English classes and a specialized program for FEPs transitioning to NPs at KSU.

Finally, the fourth common concept identified was gratefulness. Both participants, Christy and Emma, expressed gratitude in their interviews. Christy believed in God, destiny, and hard work and was grateful to finally find sanctuary in the United States from the persecution she faced in her home country. She expressed thanks to God for her life and education at KSU's nursing school as positive impacts that changed her life history. Each showed gratitude for her family's support: Christy in her caring mother and Emma in her helpful husband and children. The ability to provide healthcare and actively participate as a community member in the United States elicited many thanks and praises in both women. Convinced of divine intervention, Emma, like Christy, praised God for the opportunity provided by KSU as a miracle, a fairy tale becoming reality, thanks to him.

CONCLUSION

Even though both of the international physicians went through completely different experiences from two different cultures, there were still common themes that emerged from the interviews. Hope, discovery, challenges, and gratefulness are emotions that most humans have experienced at some point in the process of living life, especially when going through transitions. The process of being human gives way to great joys and great sorrows. The very act of living is fraught with a journey that is as personal as it is diverse in culture, ethnicity, and situations.

Even given these diversities, it was learned through the interviews of these two international physicians that the human experience can be universal. Great challenges can be overcome and foreign physicians can transition into nursing with a sense of accomplishment and profound joy. Both of these international physicians turned U.S. NPs expressed a deep and sincere thankfulness to God and the KSU nursing school for leading them through their respective journeys.

IMPLICATIONS FOR NURSING PRACTICE AND THE ROLE OF THE NP

This is an important research study for any graduate programs considering a foreign physician to NP bridge degree. This study demonstrates the importance of providing international physicians with the opportunity to translate their medical skills into practice in this country, without having to reenter physician residency. To date, very little research has been done on the subject of foreign physicians bridging over to NPs within U.S. society. Aside from KSU, only one other school in the United States offers this curriculum.

U.S. NPs work in diverse settings with multicultural collaborators and patients. It is, therefore, important to understand the great lengths that immigrant physicians have to go through in order to practice medicine in this country. Understanding this will not only give one an appreciation of the struggles faced by a fellow NP who is an immigrant but also shed light on the factors that make practicing in this country difficult for them.

RECOMMENDATIONS FOR FURTHER RESEARCH

The investigators of this research study recommend extending the investigation to include the life history of all foreign physicians who have graduated from a master's degree NP program for international physicians. In addition, they recommend an evaluation of the impact of these new NPs on their respective communities.

Finally, continued evaluation of the research is encouraged in order to study the ongoing benefit to the surrounding communities of having a bridge program for foreign physicians who transition to NPs.

COMMENTARY

From International Physician to U.S. Nurse Practitioner: Multiple Life History Study
Janice Flynn, Genie Dorman, and Mary de Chesnay

This chapter documents the case study of two foreign-born physicians (FBP) experiencing transition from foreign medical doctor in the country where the medical degree was obtained to nurse practitioner in the United States. The authors, Krisola Marcano, Charlotte Ndema, Nancy Martinez, and Jennifer Azelton, completed the research as part of the requirement for a two-semester graduate research and theory course in the WellStar Primary Care Nurse Practitioner Program at the WellStar School of Nursing (WSON), KSU. Case study methodology was used to conduct semi-structured interviews with two participants enrolled in the FBP to Nurse Practitioner Program at WSON. Three of the authors are FBP enrolled in the same class as the interviewees. In analysis, the authors identified findings that are informative and enlightening.

The participants interviewed talked about their country of origin, placing emphasis on culture, family, medical school experience, and medical practice in the country of medical education and other countries where they had lived and worked. Both participants had left their home countries and immigrated to the United States in an effort to build a better life for themselves and their families. They recounted difficulties in their country of origin, including fear of persecution and/or pressure from family members to leave and move to the United States. Both also faced significant challenges in trying to obtain a medical residency once they had settled here. The participants took and successfully passed the U.S. medical board examinations, but experienced great frustration at not being matched with a medical residency. Both had spent years seeking a residency while working at a variety of health-related jobs, such as being a nursing assistant, or other non–health-related jobs where they could not utilize their knowledge or skills. Both of the participants expressed gratitude for the opportunity afforded to them by the FBP to FNP Program, but they also reported that the program was rigorous and challenging. In addition, both noted that the transition from the role of a physician to the role of the nurse was difficult on many levels.

After analysis of transcribed interviews, the researchers grouped common themes such as discovery, perseverance, frustration, and joy. The authors also related many transitional changes for both participants, including immigration, environmental, sociocultural, and professional transitions. In the review of literature, the authors focused primarily on the mid-range Theory of Transition by Meleis (2010). The application, interpretation, and integration of multiple transitions experienced by the participants were appropriate for this applied research.

The chapter contributes much to the literature where transition from FBP to NP in the United States is rare. Currently, there are only two schools of nursing that report this type of program. The authors have identified issues that could help other schools see the value of programs of this nature and also serve as a foundation for future research.

REFERENCES

Alpert, P. T., Yucha, C. B., & Atienza, M. (2013). An advanced practice nursing program for foreign medical doctors: A practical approach. *Nursing Education Perspectives, 34*(4), 254–259. doi:10.5480/1536-5026-34.4.254

Chen, P. G.-C., Nunez-Smith, M., Bernheim, S. M., Berg, D., Gozu, A., & Curry, L. A. (2010). Professional experiences of international medical graduates practicing primary care in the United States. *Journal of General Internal Medicine, 25*(9), 947–953. doi:10.1007/s11606-010-1401-2

Flowers, M., & Olenick, M. (2014). Transitioning from physician to nurse practitioner. *Journal of Multidisciplinary Healthcare, 7*, 51–54. doi:10.2147/JMDH.S56948

Garrido, M., Simon, S. R., Purnell, L., Scisney-Matlock, M., & Pontious, S. (2016). Cultural nursing andragogies with foreign-educated physicians enrolled in BSN to MSN program. *Journal of Cultural Diversity, 23*(3), 99–105.

Goodman, J., Schlossberg, N. K., & Anderson, M. L. (2006). *Counseling adults in transition: Linking practice with theory* (3rd ed.). New York, NY: Springer Publishing.

Grossman, D., & Jorda, M. (2008). Transitioning foreign-educated physicians to nurses: The new Americans in nursing accelerated program. *Journal of Nursing Education, 47*(12), 544–551. doi:10.3928/01484834-20081201-03

Hamric, A. B., Hanson, C. M., Tracy, M. F., & O'Grady, E. T. (2014). *Advanced practice nursing: An integrative approach* (5th ed.). St. Louis, MO: Elsevier Saunders.

Iglehart, J. K. (2014). Meeting the demand for primary care: Nurse Practitioners answer the call. Retrieved from National Institute for Health

Care Management website: http://www.nihcm.org/component/content/article/6-expert-voices/1269-meeting-the-demand-for-primary-care-nurse-practitioners-answer-the-call

Jauregui, A. B., & Xu, Y. (2010). Transition into practice: Experiences of Filipino physician-turned nurse practitioners. *Journal of Transcultural Nursing, 21*(3), 257–264. doi:10.1177/1043659609358787

Levine, J. (2001). Working with victims of persecution: Lessons from Holocaust survivors. *Social Work, 46*(4), 350–360. doi:10.1093/sw/46.4.350

Libby, D. L., Zhou, Z., & Kindig, D. A. (1997). Will minority physician supply meet U.S. needs? *Health Affairs, 16*(4), 205–214. doi:10.1377/hlthaff.16.4.205

Meleis, A. I. (2010). *Transitions theory: Middle-range and situation specific theories in nursing research and practice.* New York, NY: Springer Publishing.

Meleis, A. I., Sawyer, L. M., Im, E., Hilfinger-Messias, D. K., & Schumacher, K. (2000). Experiencing transitions: An emerging middle-range theory. *Advances in Nursing Science, 23*(1), 12–28.

Meuter, R., Segalowitz, N., Hocking, J., Gallois, C., & Ryder, A. (2015). Overcoming language barriers in healthcare: A protocol for investigating safe and effective communication when patients or clinicians use a second language. *BMC Health Services Research, 15*(1), 371. doi:10.1186/s12913-015-1024-8

Neiterman, E., & Bourgeault, I. L. (2015). Professional integration as a process of professional resocialization: Internationally educated health professionals in Canada. *Social Science & Medicine, 131*, 74–81. doi:10.1016/j.socscimed.2015.02.043

Ognyanova, D., Maier, C. B., Wismar, M., Girasek, E., & Busse, R. (2012). Mobility of health professionals pre and post 2004 and 2007 EU enlargements: Evidence from the EU project PROMeTHEUS. *Health Policy, 108*(2–3), 122–132. doi:10.1016/j.healthpol.2012.10.006

Pande, V. (2014). A comparative study of reciprocity in international physician licensing. *International Journal of Pharmaceutical and Healthcare Marketing, 8*(3), 265–283. doi:10.1108/IJPHM-06-2014-0031

Peterson, B. D., Pandya, S. S., & Leblang, D. (2014). Doctors with borders: Occupational licensing as an implicit barrier to high skill migration. *Public Choice, 160*(1–2), 45–63. doi:10.1007/s11127-014-0152-8

Vapor, V. R., & Xu, Y. (2011). Double whammy for a new breed of foreign-educated nurses: Lived experiences of Filipino physician-turned nurses in the United States. *Research and Theory for Nursing Practice, 25*(3), 210–226. doi:10.1891/1541-6577.25.3.210

II

Exemplars of Health Policy in Specific Countries

Localization of the Nursing Workforce in the Sultanate of Oman

Christie Emerson

Due to rapid economic development during the past 40 years, the countries in the Arab Gulf Cooperation Council (GCC) are heavily reliant on migrant workers across all sectors of the workforce, from highly skilled professionals to unskilled laborers (Al-Riyami, Fischer, & Lopez, 2015; Zerovec & Bontenbal, 2011). In an attempt to reduce dependence on foreign labor and solve the unemployment status of nationals, GCC countries have implemented national labor policies to localize all sectors of their workforce. Localization is the process of replacing expatriate workers with nationals to decrease reliance on expatriates in the labor force (Swailes, Al Said, & Al Fahdi, 2012; Zerovec & Bontenbal, 2011).

Similar to the other countries in the Gulf region, the Sultanate of Oman has faced the problem of high domestic unemployment alongside heavy reliance on an imported workforce (Zerovec & Bontenbal, 2011). For this reason, in the early 1990s, government leaders formulated a strategic national development plan that included a focus on Omanization, the replacement of expatriate workers with Omani nationals. The healthcare workforce has been particularly dependent on skilled migrant workers due to the rapid expansion of Omani healthcare services and lack of qualified Omani healthcare professionals. In accordance with the Omanization policy, since 1990 the Ministry of Health (MoH) in Oman has expanded education and training for nurses in an attempt to increase Omanization of the nursing workforce

(Al-Riyami et al., 2015). Omanization for nurses has been higher than for physicians (Ghosh, 2009), yet the percentage of Omani nurses is still only 59% (Ministry of Health [MoH], 2014). The purpose of this chapter is to describe why localization of the nursing workforce in Oman is important, examine current policies and reports that relate to localization of the nursing workforce, and summarize the results of fieldwork activities undertaken to understand Omanization of the nursing workforce from various perspectives.

RATIONALE

The World Health Organization (WHO, 1946) constitution states that "the highest attainable standard of health is a fundamental right of every human being" (para. 1); however, equitable access to health services is impossible without an adequate supply of health workers. Campbell et al. (2013) estimated a worldwide shortage of 7.2 million health workers, with 83 countries facing a health workforce crisis. While nursing is not the only healthcare profession with a shortage, it is the most critical because nurses deliver the highest percentage of patient care at all levels and because of the immensity of the shortage of nurses (Oulton, 2006). According to Buchan and Calman (2005), the shortage of qualified nurses is one of the biggest obstacles to achieving the United Nation's (UN) Millennium Development Goals (MDG) for improving health and well-being of the global population. According to Loversidge (2016), nursing workforce regulation has a significant impact on the adequate supply of qualified nurses, and the WHO encourages member countries to enact policies to address shortages of nursing workforce (WHO, 2013).

Similar to other countries facing nursing shortages, Oman has depended on a migrant nursing workforce in order to meet the healthcare needs of the people since modernization of the healthcare system began in 1971. While nurse migration can offer mutual benefits to both source and destination countries, it also has potential negative effects on health-care in both countries. For this reason, in 2010, the WHO developed the *WHO Global Code of Practice on the International Recruitment of Health Personnel* (WHO, 2010) which states:

> Member States should strive, to the extent possible, to create a sustainable health workforce and work towards establishing effective health workforce planning, education and training, and retention strategies that will reduce their need to recruit migrant health personnel. (p. 5)

A shortage of qualified nurses affects access to quality healthcare, and while a migrant nursing workforce is a common solution, it has potential negative effects. Therefore, localization of the nursing workforce in Oman is an issue of relevance to nursing. General information about Oman, the history and structure of the Omani healthcare system, and the history of the Omani nursing workforce are provided in order to situate an examination of policies regarding Omanization of the nursing workforce.

BACKGROUND

The Sultanate of Oman, with a population of 3.6 million (WHO, 2015a), is a high-income country located in the southeast corner of the Arabian Peninsula. It is bordered by the Kingdom of Saudi Arabia and the United Arab Emirates (UAE) to the west, Yemen to the south, the Strait of Hormuz to the north, and the Arabian Sea to the east (MoH, n.d.). The median age is 26 years, with 23% under 15 years old and 4% over 60 years old. Life expectancy is 79 years for females and 75 years for males. The leading cause of death is cardiovascular disease (WHO, 2015a).

The Omani system of government is an absolute monarchy. Sultan Qaboos bin Said al Said is the monarch and head of state (Central Intelligence Agency, 2016). A renaissance in the country began when Sultan Qaboos came to power in 1970 (Al Awaisi, Cooke, & Pryjmachuk, 2015; Alshishtawy, 2010). Prior to 1970, Oman's economy was based primarily on agriculture and fishing. However, with the discovery of oil reserves, it has undergone a time of rapid economic growth (Aycan, Al-Hamadi, Davis, & Budhwar, 2007; Zerovec & Bontenbal, 2011). As described previously, this rapid growth necessitated a dependence on migrant workers in all sectors of the workforce, but by the late 1980s the government recognized the limitations that dependence on a migrant workforce would have on future development of the country. In the mid-1990s, a long-term economic development plan known as "Vision 2020" was adopted, which contained a policy for Omanization of the entire workforce (Aycan et al., 2007).

Prior to 1970, healthcare in Oman was limited and sparse, with the Oman people relying predominantly on traditional medicine. There were only two hospitals (12 beds in total), both located in Muscat, overseen by the American Mission. Only a few, mostly expatriate, physicians and nurses, with a limited number of Omani paramedic staff, ran the hospitals. Additionally, there were 10 clinics in the interior of the country staffed by healthcare assistants, with periodic visits by the Muscat hospitals' medical teams. At this time, the citizens of Oman had no other options for healthcare services (Funsch, 2015).

In 1971, the MoH was established and given responsibility for the organization and development of the National Health System of Oman. Health planning has been accomplished through a series of 5-year plans initiated in 1976. Thus far, health planning has gone through three phases. The first phase, 1976 to 1990, focused mainly on building the health infrastructure. The second phase, 1991 to 2005, focused on decentralization of the health services and the establishment of 10 health regions. Beginning in 2006, a new phase began which concentrated on disease prevention and health promotion in the community (Alshishtawy, 2010). Alongside these 5-year plans, the MoH developed a healthcare Human Resources Development Plan that focused efforts on strategies and plans for further development of healthcare human resources and for a gradual and smooth Omanization of the healthcare workforce (WHO, 2006).

At the time of the Omani renaissance in 1970, there were only five Omani nurses (Al-Riyami et al., 2015). Since that time, the MoH has established diploma nursing institutes across the country in an effort to provide students with access to nursing education opportunities in close proximity to their homes. The availability of local nursing training has significantly contributed to Omanization levels (Alshishtawy, 2010). In 1975, there were only 450 nurses working in Oman (Alshishtawy, 2010), most of whom were migrants. However, by the end of 2014, there were 14,623 working nurses, 59% of whom were Omani (MoH, 2014). There are currently nine diploma programs, two RN to BSN programs, and two university BSN programs. Additionally, the MoH has established the Oman Specialized Nursing Institute to offer post-diploma certificates in nursing specialties (MoH, 2014).

CURRENT OMANIZATION OF THE NURSING WORKFORCE POLICIES

As previously described, health planning in Oman has been accomplished through a series of 5-year plans from the MoH. The current 339-page plan describes the National Health Policy of the Sultanate of Oman; strategic directives for health development in Oman; visions, goals, and objectives of the plan; and the domains for objective achievement. As the 2016 to 2020 plan is not yet publically available, the 2011 to 2020 plan was reviewed for the most recent Omanization of the nursing workforce policies.

Goal 7 of eight total goals of the National Health Policy of the Sultanate of Oman states: "Development and training of Omani workforce in all health professional categories in order to achieve high levels of Omanization or self-sufficiency in health workforce" (MoH, Sultanate of Oman, 2011, p. 2). The following statement, located in the nursing care domain in the document, addresses how Omanization should be achieved:

> In order to speed up development processes, the Ministry has expanded in the establishment of colleges of nursing in the various governorates and regions to a total of 12 Nursing Institutes that graduate 7703 nurses up to the year 2010. Thus, the ratio of Omanization cadres had reached 66% in 2010, but exceeded 95% in some areas. For the sake of the ministry to continue to develop its human resources, it provides internal or external scholarships to some of the nursing staff to get diplomas specialist or bachelor's degree or master's in order to achieve the vision of the ministry and the needs of the required qualified staff. (MoH, Sultanate of Oman, 2011, p. 51)

This policy provides clear evidence of the priority placed by the Omani government on Omanization of the nursing workforce.

REVIEW OF THE LITERATURE

Review of the scholarly literature from the last 10 years identified issues relevant to localization of the nursing workforce in Oman. Search terms were *Oman, GCC, localization, Omanization, nursing workforce, healthcare workforce,* and *workforce.* The articles were reviewed for themes regarding effects of localization on the work environment and the impact on nursing.

There was wide variation in the disciplinary sources, methodology, and sampling of the articles. The articles reviewed were from three disciplines: business and economics (Al-Waqfi & Forstenlechner, 2010; Forstenlechner & Rutledge, 2010), health policy (Ghosh, 2009; WHO, 2015b), and nursing (Al Awaisi et al., 2015; Al-Riyami et al., 2015; Kamanyire & Achora, 2015; Shukri, Bakkar, El-Damen, & Ahmed, 2013; Wong et al., 2015). Various types of methodology were utilized in examining issues of localization. These included the following: qualitative methods using focus groups (Al-Riyami et al., 2015), case study (Al Awaisi et al., 2015; Ghosh, 2009), quantitative questionnaires (Al-Waqfi & Forstenlechner, 2010; Shukri et al., 2013), integrative literature review (Wong et al., 2015), and systematic policy review (Forstenlechner & Rutledge, 2010; WHO, 2015b).

Sampling for the qualitative and quantitative studies included both Omanis and migrants.

One theme identified in the literature was that in order for localization policies to be effective, the Omani nationals must be educated so that they have the necessary skills to assume the work currently done by migrants. Al-Waqfi and Forstenlechner (2010) concluded that in the UAE, another GCC country with similar localization policies, a lack of competence due to poor training can lead to negative stereotyping of nationals and poor relationships in the workforce. In a systematic review of WHO documents from 2007 to 2012 regarding nursing, nursing workforce issues and nurse migration were both identified as problems that need to be addressed (Wong et al., 2015). WHO (2015a, 2015b) policy recommendations included a priority that "Countries have a national nursing and midwifery workforce plan as part of the national health workforce plan" (p. 700). In a qualitative study by Al-Riyami et al. (2015), Omani nurses and Omani nursing students were interviewed about the Omanization policy. One of the themes identified in this study was that Omani nursing education must be improved for Omanis to be adequately prepared to take over for experienced migrant nurses. The Omani participants also reported the need for baccalaureate level nursing education to successfully meet the challenges of nursing work. Kamanyire and Achora (2015) also concluded that a baccalaureate degree is necessary for nurses to provide adequate nursing care.

Another theme that emerged was, that in spite of the barriers, Omanization in the health workforce should continue. Ghosh (2009) concluded that careful planning has been initiated to make improvements to the Omani healthcare workforce, and that this careful planning should continue. Shukri et al. (2013) found that both male and female students at Sultan Qaboos University had positive attitudes toward the nursing profession, and the authors recommended that policy makers continue efforts to increase awareness of the positive value of nursing so that the Omanization of the nursing workforce can continue. Al-Riyami et al. (2015) concluded that the Omani nurses and Omani students found value in Omanization but believed that the process should be slowed down. They also believed that migrant nurses were often their best mentors. Conversely, Al Awaisi et al. (2015) found that there was a tense relationship between new graduate Omani nurses and migrant nurses during their first year of practice. Forstenlechner and Rutledge (2010) suggested that localization policies could generate distrust between national and migrant workers but also believed that localization should continue.

A few articles specifically addressed Omanization of the nursing workforce (Al Awaisi et al., 2015; Al-Riyami et al., 2015; Ghosh, 2009; Kamanyire &

Achora, 2015; Shukri et al., 2013; Swailes et al., 2012). However, other articles addressed localization in other GCC countries or in the health-care workforce, but did not specify nursing (Al-Waqfi & Forstenlechner, 2014; Forstenlechner & Rutledge, 2010; WHO, 2015b; Wong et al., 2015; Zerovec & Bontenbal, 2011). There are certainly gaps in the literature on Omanization in the nursing workforce. There were no articles regarding patient perspectives of Omanization of the nursing workforce, and none that addressed patient outcomes. Other areas for further research include the perspectives of migrant nurses and nursing administrators.

FIELDWORK SUMMARY

In order to add the perspective of nurses who work in Oman to my understanding of Omanization of the nursing workforce, nurses employed in various positions at a large academic medical center in Oman were informally asked about the impact of Omanization policies on them. Additionally, nurse educators at a university college of nursing were also asked about their perspective on Omanization. The informants can be divided into the following categories: Omani nursing administrators, managers, and clinical nurse specialists (CNS); migrant nurse managers and CNS from various countries of origin; and migrant nurse educators from various countries of origin. Both male and female nurses were represented in all categories of informants.

Omani nursing administrators explained that while Omanization is a National Health Policy, the hospital had no particular policy that requires the hiring of Omani nurses. It is just understood that Omanization is the goal. Also, as the BSN is the minimum education requirement for employment, and although they would like to hire more Omani nurses, they can only recruit and retain a very few. Only 24.6% of the nursing workforce at this facility is Omani. Migrant nurses are valued and are paid the same as the Omani nurses, but the administrators know that they will eventually return to their countries of origin.

Omani nursing managers and CNS expressed that they value their migrant nurse colleagues. They believe that the migrant nurses are needed for their expertise and to train Omani nurses. Most of these nurses stated that nursing was not their first choice of study, but that they now believe that the work is important and enjoyable.

Some migrant nurse managers stated that they have been in Oman for many years (20–30 years), but they plan to return to their country of origin as required when they retire. Since most contracts are for 2 years, one migrant nurse manager said that if a migrant nurse wants to stay in Oman, they must bring something special to the workforce, be willing to work hard, and be appreciative of the opportunity to work in Oman.

According to the nurse educators, Omani students are often hard to motivate because they are not excited about nursing. There are currently no Omani nurse faculty or administrators; all are migrants. They expressed frustration at heavy workloads and frustration that they are not respected in the university community. Most believed that this perceived lack of respect was due to their migrant status and a lack of respect for nursing.

A nurse recruiter for an international nursing recruitment agency was also interviewed but did not add a new perspective on Omanization of the nursing workforce. From the informal interviews, the most common theme is that both Omani and migrant nurses understand the need for Omanization of the nursing workforce and accept it. Both respect the contributions of the other to patient care. While the Omani nurses have advantages that the migrant nurses do not, both groups believe that they work well together. Further fieldwork should include discussions with Omani and migrant patients about their views of the impact of Omanization. Further discussions with nursing administrators about safety and quality issues related to Omanization would also add important information.

SUMMARY AND CONCLUSION

Analysis of policies regarding localization of the nursing workforce in Oman indicates that it is an important issue. The Omanization policy in the National Health Policy of the Sultanate of Oman is part of the larger context of localization workforce policies in all the GCC countries and across all sectors of the workforce. The policy is also influenced by the government priority to provide quality healthcare to the people of Oman. Achieving this priority requires an adequate nursing workforce mixed with the desire for increased self-reliance. Also of importance in the analysis are the WHO recommendations regarding migration of nurses. This migration can have a negative impact on the migrating nurses' country of origin as well as on the patient care outcomes in the host country (WHO, 2010).

A review of pertinent literature reveals that there are few studies that examine localization specifically in Oman and even fewer that specifically exam localization of the nursing workforce. Although few studies target

Omanization of nursing specifically, some studies from other disciplines are generalizable to nursing. Further research is needed on the impact of Omanization of the nursing workforce on patients as well as best ways to facilitate and implement Omanization.

Perspectives gained from fieldwork in Oman show that both migrant and Omani nurses understand the need for Omanization policies. Both groups respect the contributions of the other and generally work collaboratively for the good of the patients. Further fieldwork should be done to investigate how patients view Omanization of the nursing workforce.

Efforts to localize of the nursing workforce are not unique to the Sultanate of Oman; other GCC countries are facing similar problems. Oman has experienced huge growth and many changes in a short time, but careful planning and implementation of localization policies has accomplished gradual progression toward Omanization of the nursing workforce. There is a need for continued attention to the effects of Omanization, alongside careful evaluation to make the process as smooth as possible.

REFERENCES

Al Awaisi, H., Cooke, H., & Pryjmachuk, S. (2015). The experiences of newly graduated nurses during their first year of practice in the Sultanate of Oman: A case study. *International Journal of Nursing Studies, 52*, 1723–1734. doi:10.1016/j.ijnurstu.2015.06.009

Al-Riyami, M., Fischer, I., & Lopez, V. (2015). Nurses' perceptions of the challenges related to the Omanization policy. *International Nursing Review, 62*(4), 462–469. doi:10.1111/inr.12221

Alshishtawy, M. M. (2010). Four decades of progress: Evolution of the health system in Oman. *Sultan Qaboos University Medical Journal, 10*(1), 12–22.

Al-Waqfi, M., & Forstenlechner, I. (2010). Stereotyping of citizens in an expatriate-dominated labour market: Implications for workforce localization policy. *Employee Relations, 32*(4), 364–381. doi:10.1108/01425451011051596

Al-Waqfi, M., & Forstenlechner, I. (2014). Barriers to Emiratization: The role of policy design and institutional environment in determining the effectiveness of Emiratization. *International Journal of Human Resource Management, 25*(2), 167–189. doi:10.1080/09585192.2013.826913

Aycan, Z., Al-Hamadi, A., Davis, A., & Budhwar, P. (2007). Cultural orientations and preferences for HRM policies and practices: The case of Oman.

International Journal of Human Resource Management, 18(1), 11–32. doi:10.1080/09585190601068243

Buchan, J., & Calman, L. (2005). *Summary: The global shortage of registered nurses.* Geneva, Switzerland: International Council of Nurses.

Campbell, J., Dussault, G., Buchan, J., Pozo-Martin, F., Guerra Arias, M., Leone, C., ... Comett, G. (2013). *A universal truth: No health without a workforce* (Forum Report, Third Global Forum on Human Resources for Health). Geneva, Switzerland: Global Health Workforce Alliance and World Health Organization.

Central Intelligence Agency. (Ed.). (2016). Oman. Retrieved from https://www .cia.gov/library/publications/resources/the-world-factbook/geos/mu.html

Forstenlechner, I., & Rutledge, E. (2010). Unemployment in the Gulf: Time to update the "social contract". *Middle East Policy, 17*(2), 38–51. doi:10.1111/j.1475-4967.2010.00437.x

Funsch, L. (2015). *Oman reborn: Balancing tradition and modernization.* Melbourne, Vic: Palgrave MacMillan.

Ghosh, B. (2009). Health workforce development planning in the sultanate of Oman: A case study. *Human Resources for Health, 7,* 47. doi:10.1186/1478-4491-7-47

Kamanyire, J. K., & Achora, S. (2015). A call for more diploma nurses to attain a baccalaureate degree: Advancing the nursing profession in Oman. *Sultan Qaboos University Medical Journal, 15*(3), e322–e326. doi:10.18295/ squmj.2015.15.03.004

Loversidge, J. (2016). Government regulation: Parallel and powerful. In J. Milstead (Ed.), *Health policy and politics: A nurse's guide* (5th ed., p. 32). Burlington, MA: Jones & Bartlett Learning.

Ministry of Health. (2014). Annual health report 2014. Retrieved from https:// www.moh.gov.om/en/about-oman

Ministry of Health, Sultanate of Oman. (n.d.). About Oman. Retrieved from https://www.moh.gov.om/en/about-oman

Ministry of Health, Sultanate of Oman. (2011). The 8th five-year plan for health development (2011–2015). Retrieved from https://www.mah.se/upload/ five_year_plan_for_health_development_2011-2015%20Oman.pdf

Oulton, J. A. (2006). The global nursing shortage: An overview of issues and actions. *Policy, Politics, & Nursing Practice, 7*(3), 34S–39S. doi:10.1177/1527154406293968

Shukri, R. K., Bakkar, B. S., El-Damen, M., & Ahmed, S. M. (2013). Attitudes of students at Sultan Qaboos University towards the nursing profession. *Sultan Qaboos University Medical Journal, 13*(4), 539–544. doi:10.12816/0003313

Swailes, S., Al Said, L. G., & Al Fahdi, S. (2012). Localization policy in Oman: A psychological contracting interpretation. *International Journal of Public Sector Management, 25*(5), 357–372. doi:10.1108/09513551211252387

Wong, F. K. Y., Liu, H., Wang, H., Anderson, D., Seib, C., & Molasiotis, A. (2015). Global nursing issues and development: Analysis of World Health Organization documents. *Journal of Nursing Scholarship, 47*(6), 574–583. doi:10.1111/jnu.12174

World Health Organization. (1946). *Constitution of WHO: Principles.* Geneva, Switzerland: Author. Retrieved from http://www.who.int/about/mission/en/

World Health Organization. (2006). *Health system profile: Oman.* Cairo, Egypt: Author.

World Health Organization. (2010). *The WHO global code of practice on the international recruitment of health personnel* (Sixty-third World Health Assembly, Document WHA 63.16). Geneva, Switzerland: Author.

World Health Organization. (2013). *Global health workforce shortage to reach 12.9 million in coming decades.* Geneva, Switzerland: Author. Retrieved from http://www.who.int/mediacentre/news/releases/2013/health-workforce-shortage/en/

World Health Organization. (2015a). *Oman: WHO statistical profile.* Geneva, Switzerland: Author.

World Health Organization. (2015b). *Summary report: Fourth seminar on health diplomacy.* Geneva, Switzerland: Author

Zerovec, M., & Bontenbal, M. (2011). Labor nationalization policies in Oman: Implications for Omani and migrant women workers. *Asian & Pacific Migration Journal (Scalabrini Migration Center), 20*(3), 365–387. Retrieved from http://proxy.kennesaw.edu/login?url=http://search.ebscohost.com/login.aspx?direct=true&db=sih&AN=71342443&site=eds-live&scope=site

Perspectives of Culture and Chronic Disease in the United Arab Emirates

Jennifer Cooper
Sharon Brownie

The United Arab Emirates (UAE) is a rapidly developing country comprised of a multinational population with varying educational backgrounds, cultural practices, and religious beliefs (Loney et al., 2013). Impacted by social and environmental factors, the built environment and contemporary lifestyles pose major public health challenges to this modern Arab and expatriate world with noncommunicable (NCD) and chronic disease an increasing concern. The aforementioned challenges significantly contribute to morbidity and mortality in the UAE (Rahim et al., 2014). NCD and chronic disease is not isolated to the UAE alone, but forms part of a global health crisis, requiring international global health policy, collaboration, and action (Hajat, Harrison, & Shather, 2012).

CONTEXT

Comprised of seven Emirates, the UAE is situated southeast of the Arabian Peninsula, sharing borders with Oman and Saudi Arabia (Loney et al., 2013). This small, newly formed nation is known for its involvement in world trade and its modern industrial progress. A 1995 national census reported a total UAE population of 2.7 million, with 20% UAE nationals (National Census, 1995). The remainder of the population was from India, Pakistan, East Asia, and Europe (National Census, 1995). Twenty-year growth to 2015 estimates a total population increase to 9.7 million, with a total of 13% UAE nationals (UAE National Bureau of Statistics, 2015).

The UAE has experienced and continues to experience rapid changes in economic development and urbanization with significant impact on lifestyle behaviors and culture (Alhyas, McKay, & Majeed, 2012). These lifestyle changes have caused an increase in NCDs such as cardiovascular disease, cancers, respiratory disease, and type 2 diabetes. Risk factors for these diseases, such as tobacco use, physical inactivity, and an unhealthy diet, have also increased and led to a rise in obesity and hypertension within the UAE and the wider Arabian Gulf Region (Arab, 2003).

TRADITIONAL CULTURE AND FAITH

Culture assists in specifying which behaviors, beliefs, and practices are acceptable in a society. The differences among cultures, beliefs, and practices influence an individual and population, groups, lifestyle, and health behaviors. Culture influences social institutions, social groups, and, in turn, individuals, population health, and illness (Jirojwong & Liamputtong, 2012).

Prior to 1971, the UAE did not exist as a country and was known as the coast of Oman (Al-Fahim, 1995). In the 1800s, it was known as the Trucial states and the locals lived a Bedouin lifestyle on the land; or, they lived by the sea, where pearling and sea diving were their main forms of trade (Al-Fahim, 1995). The Bedouins lived in encampments in the desert or by the sea, and each area of Bedouins belonged to a specific tribe which had its own traditions and customs; their identity was associated with either their desert or sea existence (Al-Fahim, 1995). In the 1800s, the British made truce agreements with the leaders of the Trucial states and withdrew these agreements in 1971 (Al-Fahim, 1995). In 1971, the six Trucial states agreed on a federal constitution as an independent country now known as the UAE (Al-Fahim, 1995). At this time, the staple food consisted of dates, camel milk, and fish (Al-Fahim, 1995). The cultural traditions were adhered to, including no alcohol and pork, with meat required to be slaughtered in Islamic Halal style (World Culture Encyclopedia, 2017).

The Islamic religion is the cornerstone for all Muslims and is the religion followed by most of the population in the UAE (Central Intelligence

Agency, 2005). The Islamic faith involves submitting oneself to God and following the five pillars of Islam.

The five pillars of Islam include the following:

Shahadah: Reciting the Muslim faith

Salat: Performing prayers five times a day

Zakat: Proving monetary assistance to the poor and less fortunate than oneself

Sawm: Fasting throughout the holy month of Ramadan

Hajj: Completing the pilgrimage to Mecca once in a lifetime.

In the UAE, the official language is Arabic; however, English is the language of commerce and social service delivery. In the 1950s and early 1960s, before the discovery of oil, UAE nationals consumed and bought only necessities; however, with the discovery of oil and globalization, a Western lifestyle has resulted in evolving cultural changes. Rapid changes can bring about challenges in individual health and population health which impact social, cultural, and environmental characteristics.

The Emirati culture is known for its hospitality and socializing with friends and family. Most guests are greeted with coffee and dates (World Culture Encyclopedia, 2017) and the main meal shared with the family is the daytime meal. At large social gatherings, food is generously shared and is part of socialization. The importance of sharing food together is a vital component of the Emirati culture (Brownie, 2015). Food consumption is heavily influenced by changes in food availability in the UAE (Boutayeb et al., 2012). Despite the many changes influenced by globalization, the traditions among family within the UAE culture remain of vital importance to the lifestyle of UAE nationals. UAE nationals are heavily influenced by family; conformity and commitment to the group are paramount (Vel, Captain, Al-Abbas, & Al-Hashemi, 2011).

Culture also influences an individual or population group's health behavior, perception of health and health maintenance, response to an illness, and the type of care they seek (Huff & Kline, 1999; Kleinman, 1980). The effect culture has on population health is influenced by the complexities of the cultural, biological, social, and psychological challenges which impact on chronic disease prevention, management, and premature death.

MODERN CULTURE AND FAITH

The UAE is one of the most diverse countries in the Gulf Corporation Council (GCC), attracting many foreign investors and many expatriates, which has influenced traditional culture and values (Potter, 2011). The country is a major modern metropolis featuring five-star hotels, lavish shopping malls, and cuisine from all over the world (Potter, 2011). The older UAE nationals will recall a rural environment, while the younger generation is familiar and comfortable living in a modern, urban, and Westernized society. Western influences have influenced Arabic dress, entertainment, and marriage (Benesh, 2008). In some Arabic families, partners can be chosen instead of an arranged marriage. There is also support and acceptance for Arabic women to be educated and join the workforce (Khelifa, 2010). These changes have been the result of significant societal changes due to economic development, the promotion of higher education, and the desire to create a strong workforce of both male and female UAE nationals. However, despite the Westernized influences, fundamental values such as the influences of traditional society, culturally defined dress, the Islamic faith, and the importance of family remain a constant guiding force which affect behavior and actions (Al-Khazraji, 2009).

IMPACT AND CONSIDERATION FOR HEALTH

RISK FACTORS

Although there have been positive changes in the UAE's thriving and modern society, some changes have brought about challenges to the health status of its population. The contemporary lifestyle of UAE nationals is characterized by poor diet, high tobacco use (24% males), and physical inactivity with an associated high BMI average of 29 kg/m^2 across the UAE total population (Hajet et al., 2012). Risk factors contributing to the health status of the UAE population and increasing the risk of developing NCD and chronic diseases are outlined below.

Tobacco Use

One of the main risk factors contributing to the development of respiratory disease in the UAE is tobacco use. According to Hajet et al. (2012), "smoking rates are very high in young National males, with 16% of 18- to 20-year-olds, 27% of 20- to 29-year-olds and 28% of 30- to 39-year-olds" being smokers, but less than 1% of women smoke. The smoking rates are also high among non-national males as they predominantly originate from Southeast Asia and India, which also have high rates of smoking (Health Authority Abu Dhabi Statistics Report, 2014). There are also many misconceptions about the safety of the use of the tobacco pipe (*shisha*) and Midwakh, which are both common practices of smoking throughout the Gulf region, but particularly in the UAE (Akl et al., 2010; Jayakumary, Jayadevan, Ranade, & Mathew, 2010; Kandela, 2000; Maziak, Eissenberg, & Ward, 2005). According to the Global Youth Tobacco Survey, tobacco pipe use among the 13- to 15-year-old age group has risen from 18% in 2002 to 29% in 2005 (Vupputuri et al., 2016). In children aged between 13 and 15 years who participated in the Global Youth Tobacco Survey, 82% had tried a cigarette before the age of 14 years (Vupputuri et al., 2016). These alarming statistics require utmost attention from the public health sector and offer a challenging environment for the promotion tobacco control.

Culture and cultural habits are determinants that impact this population group. Smoking among males and some females in the UAE is a habit enjoyed with friends and family (Islam & Johnson, 2003). It is a social and cultural norm and is seen as part of the country's cultural hospitality (Chaouachi, 2000).

Physical Inactivity

Physical inactivity increases the risk of NCD, including cardiovascular disease, type 2 diabetes, cancers, and respiratory disease. Physical inactivity and sedentary lifestyles have been identified as the fourth leading risk factor for mortality globally (World Health Organization [WHO], 2017).

In 2012, as part of the Lancet physical activity series working group, the effects of physical inactivity on major NCDs worldwide were reviewed as part of an analysis of the burden of disease and life expectancy (Lee et al., 2012). Physical inactivity was found to be attributable to 6% of the burden of disease from coronary heart disease, 10% of breast and colon cancer, and 7% of type 2 diabetes (Lee et al., 2012). Inactivity contributes to mortality, and if there was a 10% to 25% increase in physical activity, it is estimated that the average life expectancy across the world's population would increase by 0.68 to 0.95 years (Lee et al., 2012). Physical activity is essential for healthy lifestyles, self-efficacy, sportsmanship, and a reduction in developing risk factors for preventable lifestyle diseases such as obesity and type 2 diabetes (Bailey, 2006).

Food Consumption/Unhealthy Diet

The rapid environmental changes of urbanization and the availability, affordability, and accessibility of fast food have affected overall food consumption (Loney et al., 2013). Some of the traditional foods of the UAE included meats such as chicken, lamb, mutton, and fowl, while rice was introduced to the traditional diet when traders moved to the region. Cheese, dates, and eggs were also staples in the traditional diet, with camels being used to transport camel milk. The meat, rice, and spice dishes originate from Saudi Arabia but are also an original staple of the traditional Emirati diet, alongside coffee shared with houseguests, family, and friends (Al-Fahim, 1995).

Fast food is consumed at least once a week and sometimes daily by residents of the UAE (Rizvi & Bell, 2015). According to the YouGov health survey conducted in 2015 with UAE nationals and expatriates ($n = 1,030$; $m = 646$ and $f = 385$), 7% ordered fast food or ate out of the home daily (Rizvi & Bell, 2015) and 30% consumed fast food and/or ate out once a week (Rizvi & Bell, 2015). Poor nutrition and a consumption of high fat foods increase the risk factors for NCD and chronic diseases (WHO, 2013).

NONCOMMUNICABLE AND CHRONIC DISEASE IN THE UAE

NCD and chronic diseases are the world's biggest killers. According to the World Health Organization (WHO), 36 million individuals die annually from NCDs (WHO, 2013). By working with individuals, communities, and populations, risk factors associated with NCD and chronic diseases can be reduced. Influencing public health policy is vital to addressing risk factors, particularly those that impact long-term health outcomes for the UAE population and globally (WHO, 2013).

CARDIOVASCULAR DISEASE

Cardiovascular disease is one of the main causes of death in the UAE (Health Authority Abu Dhabi, 2011). In 2000, the WHO created a document on the global burden of disease of which, for the UAE, the main noncommunicable issues of concern were cancer, cardiovascular disease, type 2 diabetes, high mean BMI, and high rates of smoking among males (WHO, 2000). In response to this report, in 2008, the Health Authority in the Emirate of Abu Dhabi developed a screening program called Weqaya (*Weqaya* is the Arabic word for protection; Hajat et al., 2012). Ninety-four percent of the adult national population in the Emirate of Abu Dhabi were screened, and of those screened, there were extremely high levels of obesity, type 2 diabetes, prediabetes, hypertension, and high rates of tobacco use (Hajat et al., 2012). During 2008 to 2009, 17% were diagnosed with hypertension and 36% with high lipids ("Weqaya Sample," 2008).

CANCERS

The worldwide burden of cancer is reported to be rising due in part to the growth and age of the global population, and an increasing Westernized lifestyle, including the risk factors for NCD and chronic disease, as discussed earlier, tobacco use, physical inactivity, and unhealthy diets.

Cancer is the third leading cause of death in the UAE among both UAE nationals and expatriates (Statistics Centre Abu Dhabi, 2010). The leading cause of cancer-related death in males is lung cancer and breast cancer in females (Statistics Centre Abu Dhabi, 2015). In 2015, in the Emirate of Abu Dhabi, 14.1% of deaths resulted from lung cancer and 12.2% from breast cancer (Statistics Centre Abu Dhabi, 2015). Other common cancers among men in the UAE are colorectal, liver, leukemia, and pancreatic. Irrespective of breast cancer, the other most common cancers among women in the UAE are colorectal, leukemia, ovarian, and lung cancer (Statistics Centre Abu Dhabi, 2015).

Culture plays a major part in the response to signs and symptoms of illness and potential cancer diagnosis. Many UAE nationals present themselves late to healthcare facilities for treatment due to cultural and religious beliefs, fear, stigma, and family attitude toward treatment (Silbermann et al., 2013). An individual's health beliefs and practices are influenced heavily by the sociocultural environment that surrounds them, including family and friends, community and society (Assaf, Holroyd, & Lopez, 2017).

The UAE has recently developed a cancer registry; however, the data are only inclusive of public government hospitals and do not include private hospitals (Rizvi, 2017). The Ministry of Health and Prevention is developing a new National Cancer Index which will allow monitoring and surveillance of the various types of cancers and a greater understanding of the cancers affecting the UAE population (Rizvi, 2017). The burden of cancer could be reduced through early detection and treatment and public health campaigns to promote smoking cessation, physical activity, and healthy dietary intake.

RESPIRATORY DISEASE

The UAE population is at an increased risk of developing respiratory diseases due to the high incidence of tobacco use, indoor and outdoor air pollution, and extreme weather variations including major dust storms and in some cases genetics (Webster, 2016). The burden of respiratory diseases varies throughout the UAE; however, asthma, respiratory infections, sleep disorders, and chronic obstructive pulmonary disease (COPD) remain the most prevalent respiratory conditions. According to the WHO, the main factors contributing to respiratory diseases such as COPD include tobacco smoke indoor and outdoor air pollution, and exposure to occupational chemicals and dust (Webster, 2016).

Asthma is a chronic respiratory disease increasing globally, including the UAE. In the GCC region, there is inter and intraregional variability in asthma prevalence. In Oman, the prevalence varied between 7.8% and 17.3% in different regions of the country (Al-Rawas, Al-Riyami, Al-Kindy, Al-Maniri, & Al-Riyami, 2008), and in Qatar the prevalence was 19.8% (Janahi, Bener, & Bush, 2006). In Saudi Arabia, the prevalence was 23.6% (Nahhas, Bhopal, Anandan, Elton, & Sheikh, 2012). A study from Al Ain in the UAE illustrates an asthma prevalence of 13% using the International Study of Asthma and Allergies in Childhood (ISAAC) questionnaire (Al-Rawas et al., 2008), while another based on the European Community Respiratory Health Survey (ECRHS) questionnaire shows a range of 8% to 10% across the UAE (Alsowaidi, Abdulle, & Bernsen, 2010).

There has also been a rise in other respiratory diseases in the UAE, such as tuberculosis and pneumonia. According to Health Authority Abu Dhabi (HAAD), there has been evidence of rising cases of tuberculosis (TB). In the Emirate of Abu Dhabi in 2010, 450 cases of pulmonary TB and 175 cases of extrapulmonary TB were registered (El Shammaa, 2011; Qabbani, 2011).

Pneumonia is a health problem that mainly affects children under the age of 5 years and adults over 65 years. However, figures from the WHO show that 5% of deaths among children under the age of 5 years in the UAE are caused by pneumonia (Howidi, Muhsin, & Rajah, 2011).

TYPE 2 DIABETES

The modern epidemic of type 2 diabetes and its association with the rising prevalence of obesity are well established. The WHO predicts doubling the number of individuals with type 2 diabetes in the world between the years 2000 and 2025. According to the International Diabetes Federation (IDF), the UAE has the second highest incidence of diabetes in the world and many of the neighboring Gulf countries are in the top eight countries in the world with the highest rates of type 2 diabetes (International Diabetes Federation [IDF], 2011).

Type 2 diabetes usually occurs due to environmental and sometimes genetic factors; however, the risk of developing type 2 diabetes is substantially increased due to lifestyle risk factors, such as insufficient physical activity and poor diet. It is often associated with individuals who are overweight, obese, and have hypertension (Diabetes Australia, 2015).

Type 2 diabetes can often be prevented by maintaining a healthy lifestyle including a healthy diet and physical activity. However, most individuals need some form of medication to assist in disease management and to help minimize long-term complications (Bate & Jerums, 2003).

INTERPRETIVE MODEL: SOCIO-ECOLOGICAL MODEL

The socio-ecological model was originally developed in the 1970s and became a formalized theory in the 1980s. The model is used for human development to improve the understanding of the interaction between genetics and biology. Its original focus was on children (Bronfenbrenner, 1989). The model continued to be revised to include the interrelatedness of the physical and social environment and the impact this has on an individual's attitudes and beliefs (Bronfenbrenner, 1989).

The socio-ecological model illustrates the interaction between an individual, community, and society and where individual behaviors are influenced by multiple factors. An individual is influenced by family,

family history, and genetics. Communities such as schools, workplaces, and neighborhoods also impact an individual's behavior and attitude, while the broader society influences an individual's social and cultural norms (McLeroy, Bibeau, Steckler, & Glanz, 1998). For behavior change to be instilled, culture, environment, and government policies need to be aligned (Caprio et al., 2008).

The socio-ecological model illustrates five levels that influence an individual's behavior: individual, interpersonal, community, organization, and policy (Bronfenbrenner, 1993). Each level intersects and connects with the others so that an individual's knowledge, values, beliefs, and self-efficacy are influenced by many factors, such as family and friends (interpersonal), access to information and social capital (community), and resources and services (Bronfenbrenner, 1993).

INDIVIDUAL

The individual is situated in the center of the social-ecological model. This level includes personal factors that increase or decrease the likelihood of an individual making behavioral changes (Bronfenbrenner, 1989). Individual influences include an individual's age, gender, education level, socioeconomic status, and self-efficacy. It also includes an individual's knowledge, attitudes, behaviors, beliefs, barriers, and motivation (Bronfenbrenner, 1989).

There is a complex interplay between individual behaviors, cultural influences, and environmental factors that is represented by the socio-ecological model which illustrates the multiple factors that influence behavior (Townsend & Foster, 2011). Human behaviors, including participation in physical activity, decreasing tobacco use, and consuming a healthy diet, are improved when an individual's environment supports healthy choices. The socio-ecological model acknowledges that it requires a combination of individual, environmental, and policy-level interventions to achieve sustainable changes in health behaviors.

INTERPERSONAL

The interpersonal environment comprises the relationships between family and friends, and an individual's culture and values, and the society in which an individual interacts (Bronfenbrenner, 1989). The interpersonal environment has a significant influence on an individual's behavior. If an individual is surrounded by family and friends who participate in physical activity and healthy food choices, this can impact the behavior of others (Bronfenbrenner, 1989).

The socio-ecological model helps to explain the relationships between the constructs of family and cultural norms: their expectations and obligations being integral to lifestyle, irrespective of the severity of an individual's NCD or chronic disease. An individual's beliefs, attitudes, and behavior are impacted and influenced by cultural norms and expectations, cultural identity, and the wider community (Bronfenbrenner, 1989).

COMMUNITY

The community context in which social relationships are developed include environments such as schools, neighborhoods, and workplaces. Community also incorporates parks and recreation utilized for leisure time with family and friends (Jirojwong & Liamputtong, 2012). The community level of the socio-ecological model supports and illustrates an individual's interactions with his or her physical and sociocultural environments (Jirojwong & Liamputtong, 2012). To reduce sedentary lifestyles and promote healthy lifestyles, all levels of the socio-ecological model need to be addressed.

Many environmental and social determinants of health have contributed to and continue to have an impact on the development of NCD and chronic diseases (Keheler and MacDougall, 2009). In the UAE, environmental determinants such as mass urbanization, a rapid increase in population size, and adverse weather conditions such as dust and sandstorms all contribute to an individual's health management (Loney et al., 2013). A lack of health knowledge and awareness, a lack of social support (most of the UAE population are living away from home), addiction, and stress are also environmental impacts that contribute to the development of NCD and chronic diseases (Jarvis, 2002). The financial accessibility and low cost of tobacco and fast food are also contributing factors (Daniel, Cargo, & Lifshay, 2004). For behavior change to occur, an individual requires a supportive community, incorporating environments that influence active living, healthy food options, and a reduction in tobacco consumption.

Community-level change can take time and requires a socio-ecological approach recognizing the complexity of factors at various levels, including the community, family, and society. Positive community-level change requires a foundation grounded in relevant cultural concepts, cultural engagement, and self-determination (Jirojwong & Liamputtong, 2012).

The UAE government authorities are aware of the need to address NCD and chronic diseases and their associated risk factors and have been actively promoting public health initiatives, particularly in schools (Regional Consultation, 2010). However, there is a continued need to increase education and awareness among the UAE population through multiparty strategies and awareness campaigns on the impact and long-term health effects of consuming high fat food and a lack of physical activity (Swan, 2017).

ORGANIZATIONAL

Individual behavioral change is influenced by organizational environments, systems, and policies (Robinson, 2008). The organizational level of the socio-ecological model overlaps with the community and policy levels and represents a vital component of the model incorporating organizations such as work environments, social institutions, healthcare and faith organizations. All individual interactions with any organizational environment influence an individual's food behavior, physical activity levels, and tobacco use (Robinson, 2008). Organizational environments are required to determine organizational systems and policies to implement strategies to support healthy lifestyle choices (Robinson, 2008).

POLICY

Policy refers to legislation and policy making carried out by local, state, or federal governments. There can also be local policies for schools, healthcare facilities, and academic institutions. Some examples of policies that can impact an individual's behavior to make healthy choices include urban planning, transport, and education policies ensuring physical activity and healthy food options are available in schools. Environmental and workplace policies also play a part in individual and community behavior change (Langille & Rodgers, 2010). Policies provide the opportunity for governments to collaborate with various organizations to promote strategies to align with healthy lifestyles and reduce risk factors for NCD and chronic diseases (Langille & Rodgers, 2010).

HEALTH WORKFORCE IMPACT

The UAE population includes a unique mix of UAE nationals, expatriates, and a large male labor workforce (Hunter, Robb, & Brownie, 2014). The UAE government relies heavily on expatriate workers; however, this reliance is changing and much of the workforce development and capacity-building has been tailored to the employment of local UAE nationals to ensure healthcare delivery can be undertaken by UAE nationals (Brownie, Lebogo, & Hag-Ali, 2014). Workforce development has been supported by local universities offering medical, nursing, and allied health degrees (Brownie et al., 2014). Due to the rapid changes in urbanization, poor dietary intake, and physical inactivity, the UAE is burdened with high rates of NCDs and chronic diseases which are challenging for the current workforce to provide appropriate healthcare services (Brownie et al., 2014).

The UAE population data sets are also difficult to ascertain given that the most recent data were published in 2010 with the latest census data based on figures from 2005 (Hunter et al., 2014). Gaps in population data and reliable health data also make it difficult for universities and healthcare services alike to provide appropriate healthcare services to meet the needs and demands of this multinational population (Brownie et al., 2014). Through the promotion of health policy and legislation, development of early detection strategies, ongoing surveillance, and an increase in health expenditure, an overall reduction in NCDs and chronic diseases could be achieved (Brownie et al., 2014).

CONCLUSION

For a reduction in NCD and chronic disease to be achieved among those living in the UAE, there needs to be a multinational, multisectorial approach, with commitment from all sector stakeholders. Healthcare education and awareness campaigns need to address the risk factors and be culturally sensitive to the needs of the population group. Education needs to be targeted at high-risk groups and be implemented in areas where the groups are easily reached, such as schools, universities, healthcare facilities, and labor camps. A country-wide cancer registry inclusive of all sectors and a surveillance program for all UAE residents need to be developed to gain a better understanding of the size of the NCD and chronic disease problems and to aid in the development of appropriate legislation and policies. The social, environmental, and cultural determinants need to be encompassed in all education, policies, and strategies to aid in the reduction of NCDs and chronic diseases. Policy makers and government departments, in collaboration with both public and private healthcare sectors and education institutions, are required to address the needs of this unique multicultural, multinational population group. The socio-ecological model represents a comprehensive approach to the design, implementation, and evaluation of health interventions which target multiple influences on behavior including the risk factors for NCDs and chronic diseases.

REFERENCES

Akl, E., Gaddam, S., Gunukula, S., Honeine, R., Abou Jaoude, P., & Irani, J. (2010). The effects of water pipe tobacco smoking on health out-comes: A systematic review. *International Journal of Epidemiology, 39*(3), 834–857. doi:10.1093/ije/dyq002

Al-Fahim, M. (1995). *From Rags to Riches: A story of Abu Dhabi.* London, UK: London Center of Arab Studies Ltd.

Alhyas, L., McKay, A., & Majeed, A. (2012). Prevalence of type 2 diabetes in the states of the co-operation council for the Arab States of the Gulf: A systematic review. *PLoS One, 7*(8), e40948. doi:10.1371/journal.pone.0040948

Al-Khazraji, N. (2009). *The culture of commercialism: Globalization in the UAE.* Washington, DC: Georgetown University.

Al-Rawas, O., Al-Riyami, B., Al-Kindy, H., Al-Maniri, A., & Al-Riyami, A. (2008). Regional variation I the prevalence of asthma symptoms among Omani school children: Comparisons from two nationwide cross-sectional surveys six years apart. *Sultan Qaboos University Medical Journal, 8*(2), 157–164.

Alsowaidi, S., Abdulle, A., & Bernsen, R. (2010). Prevalence and risk factors of asthma among adolescents and their parents in Al-Ain (United Arab Emirates). *Respiration, 79*(2), 105–111. doi:10.1159/000219248

Arab, M. (2003). The economics of diabetes care in the Middle East. In K. Alberti, P. Zimmet, & R. Defronzo (Eds.), *International textbook of diabetes mellitus* (2nd ed.). Chichester, UK: Wiley and Sons.

Assaf, G., Holyroyd, E., & Lopez, V. (2017). Isolation and prayer as a means of solace for Arab women with breast cancer: An in-depth interview study. *Psycho-Oncology, 26*(11), 1888–1893. doi:10.1002/pon.4402

Bailey, R. (2006). Physical education and sport in schools: A review of benefits and outcomes. *Journal of School Health, 76*(8), 397–401. doi:10.1111/j.1746-1561.2006.00132.x

Bate, K., & Jerums, G. (2003). Preventing complications of diabetes. *Medical Journal of Australia, 179*(9), 498–503.

Benesh, G. (2008). *Culture Shock! UAE: A survival guide to customs and etiquette.* South East Asia: Marshall Cavendish International Asia.

Boutayeb, A., Lamlili, M., Boutayeb, W., Maamri, A., Ziyyat, A., & Ramdani, N. (2012). The rise of diabetes prevalence in the Arab region. *Open Journal of Epidemiology, 2,* 55–60. doi:10.4236/ojepi.2012.22009

Bronfenbrenner, U. (1989). Ecological systems theory. In R. Vasta (Ed.), *Annals of child development* (pp. 187–249). London, UK: Jessica Kingsley.

Bronfenbrenner, U. (1993). The ecology of cognitive development: Research models and fugitive findings. In N. R. H. Wozniak & K. Fischer (Eds.), *Scientific Environments* (pp. 3–44). Hillsdale, NJ: Erlbaum.

Brownie, S. (2015). New traditions in Middle Eastern hospitality. *The Lancet Diabetes and Endocrinology, 3*(4), 304. doi:10.1016/S2213-8587(14)70254-2

Brownie, S., Lebogo, N., & Hag-Ali, M. (2014). Health care for all: Building a public health workforce to achieve the UAE 2021 vision for health. *Arab Health, 2,* 1–6.

Caprio, S., Daniels, S., Drewnowski, A., Kaufman, F., Palinkas, L., Rosenbloom, A., … Kirkman, S. (2008). Influence of race, ethnicity, and culture on childhood obesity: Implications for prevention and treatment. *Diabetes Care, 31*(11), 2211–2221. doi:10.2337/dc08-9024

Central Intelligence Agency. (2005). The world fact book—country comparison to the world. Retrieved from https://www.cia.gov/library/publications/the-world-factbook/geos/ae.html

Chaouachi, K. (2000). *Narghile (hookah): A socio-anthropological analysis. culture, conviviality, history and tobaccology of a popular tobacco use mode.* Paris, France: Universite Paris X.

Daniel, M., Cargo, M., & Lifshay, J. (2004). Cigarette smoking, mental health and social support: Data from a northwestern First Nation. *Canadian Journal of Public Health, 95,* 45–49.

Diabetes Australia. (2015). Type 2 diabetes. Retrieved from http://www.diabetesaustralia.com.au/type-2-diabetes

El Shammaa, D. (2011, May 26). Abu Dhabi implements new standards in combating TB. *Gulf News*, p. 1.

Hajat, C., Harrison, O., & Shather, Z. (2012). A profile and approach to chronic disease in Abu Dhabi. *Globalization and Health, 8*, 18. doi:10.1186/1744-8603-8-18

Health Authority Abu Dhabi. (2011). Health Statistics, 2010. Retrieved from http://www.haad.ae

Health Authority Abu Dhabi. (2014). Health Statistics, 2010. Retrieved from http://www.haad.ae

Howidi, M., Muhsin, H., & Rajah, J. (2011). The burden of pneumococcal disease in children less than 5 years of age in Abu Dhabi, United Arab Emirates. *Annals of Saudi Medicine, 31*(4), 356–359. doi:10.4103/0256-4947.83214

Huff, R. M., & Kline, M. V. (1999). Health promotion in the context of culture. In R. M. Huff, M. V. Kline, D. V. Peterson, & L. W. Green (Eds.), *Promoting health in multicultural populations: A handbook for practitioners* (pp. 3–22). Thousand Oaks, CA: SAGE Publications.

Hunter, L. H., Robb, W. F., & Brownie, S. M. (2014). The "secret" impact of population statistics on the metrics of diabetes. *Journal of Diabetes and Metabolic Disorders, 1*(4), 00024. doi:10.15406/jdmdc.2014.01. 00024

International Diabetes Federation, Diabetes Atlas. (2011). Middle East and North Africa (MENA). Retrieved from http://www.idf.org/diabetesatlas/5e/middle-east-atlas

Islam, S. M., & Johnson, C. A. (2003). Correlates of smoking behavior among Muslim Arab-American adolescents. *Ethnicity and Health, 8*, 319–337. doi:10.1080/13557850310001631722

Janahi, I., Bener, A., & Bush, A. (2006). Prevalence of asthma among Qatari school children: International Study of Asthma and Allergies in Childhood, Qatar. *Pediatric Pulmonology, 41*(1), 80–86. doi:10.1002/ppul.20331

Jarvis, M. (2002). Smoking and stress. In S. Stansfeld & M. Marmot (Eds.), *Stress and the heart*. London, UK: BMJ Books.

Jayakumary, M., Jayadevan, S., Ranade, A. V., & Mathew, E. (2010) Prevalence and pattern of Dokha use among medical and allied health students in Ajman, UAE. *Asian Pacific Cancer Journal Cancer Prevalence, 11*, 1547–1549.

Jirojwong, S., & Liamputtong, P. (2012). *Population health, communities and health promotion*. Melbourne, Australia: Oxford University Press.

Kamal-ud-Din, K. (2010). *Five pillars of Islam*. Forlag: Nabu Press.

Kandela, P. (2000). Nargille smoking keeps Arabs in wonderland. *Lancet, 356,* 1175. doi:10.1016/S0140-6736(05)72871-3

Keheler, H., & MacDougall, C. (2009). *Understanding health: A determinants approach* (2nd ed.). South Melbourne, Australia: Oxford University Press.

Khelifa, M. (2010). Trading culture: Have Western-educated Emirati females gone Western? *OIDA International Journal of Sustainable Development, 1*(3), 19–29.

Kleinman, A. (1980). *Patients and healers in the context of culture: An exploration of the borderland between anthropology, medicine, and psychiatry* (Vol. 3). Berkeley: University of California Press.

Langille, J., & Rogers, W. (2010). Exploring the influence of a social ecological model on school based physical activity. *Health Promotion Practice, 37*(6), 879–894. doi:10.1177/1090198110367877

Lee, I., Shiroma, E., Lobelo, F., Puska, P., Blair, S., & Katzmarzyk, P. (2012). Effect of physical activity on major non-communicable disease worldwide: An analysis of burden of disease and life expectancy. *Lancet, 380*(9838), 219–229. doi:10.1016/S0140-6736(12)61031-9

Loney, T., Ching-Aw, T., Handysides, D., Ali, R., Blair, I., Grivna, M., ... El-Obaid, Y. (2013). An analysis of the health status of the United Arab Emirates: The big 4 public health issues. *Global Health Action, 6,* 1–9. doi:10.3402/gha.v6i0.20100

Maziak, W., Eissenberg, T., & Ward, K. D. (2005). Patterns of water pipe use and dependence: Implications for intervention development. *Pharmacology, Biochemistry and Behavior, 80,* 173–179. doi:10.1016/j.pbb.2004.10.026

McLeroy, K., Bibeau, D., Steckler, A., & Glanz, K. (1998). An ecological perspective on health promotion programs. *Health Education Quarterly, 15*(4), 351–377. doi:10.1177/109019818801500401

Nahhas, M., Bhopal, R., Anandan, C., Elton, R., & Sheikh, A. (2010). Prevalence of allergic disorders among primary school aged children in Madinah, Saudi Arabia: Two-stage cross-sectional survey. *PLoS One, 7*(5), e36848. doi:10.1371/journal.pone.0036848

National Census. (1995). Retrieved from https://en.wikipedia.org/wiki/Demographics_of_the_United_Arab_ Emirates

Potter, L. (2011). From traditional to modern states. *Pro Quest Document Preview, 333–334,* 13–28.

Qabbani, B. (2011, September 18). Tuberculosis increases sharply among migrants. *The National.* Retrieved from https://www.thenational.ae/uae

Rahim, H., Sibai, A., Khader, Y., Hwalla, N., Fadhil, I., Alsiyabi, H., ... Husseini, A. (2014). Non-communicable diseases in the Arab world. *Lancet, 383*(9914), 356–367. doi:10.1016/S0140-6736(13)62383-1

Regional Consultation. (2010). *Regional consultation in the Eastern Mediterranean Region on the prevention and control of non-communicable diseases.* Tehran, Iran: World Health Organisation.

Rizvi, A. (2017, February 22). National cancer registry for UAE will help reduce fatalities, doctors say. *The National.* Retrieved from https://www.thenational .ae/uae

Rizvi, A., & Bell, J. (2015, January 14). UAE residents eat fast food on regular basis, YouGov survey finds. *The National.* Retrieved from https://www .thenational.ae/uae

Robinson, T. (2008). Applying the socio-ecological model to improving fruit and vegetable intake among low-income African Americans. *Journal of Community Health, 33*(6), 395–406. doi:10.1007/s10900-008-9109-5

Silbermann, M., Epner, D., Charalambous, H., Baider, L., Puchalalski, C., Balducci, L., & Smith, T. (2013). Promoting new approaches for cancer care in the Middle East. *Annals of Oncology, 24*(Suppl 7), vii5–vii10. doi:10.1093/ annonc/mdt267

Statistics Centre Abu Dhabi. (2010). Health Statistics. Retrieved from http:// www.haad.ae

Swan, M. (2017). Intervention needed to improve health of young UAE. *The National.* Retrieved from https://www.thenational.ae/uae

Townsend, N., & Foster, C. (2011). Developing and applying a socio-ecological model to the promotion of healthy eating in the school. *Public Health Nutrition, 16*(6), 1101–1108. doi:10.1017/S1368980011002655

UAE National Bureau of Statistics. (2015). Methodology of estimating the population in UAE. Retrieved from www.dubaifaqs.com/population-of-uae.php

Vel, K., Captain, A., Al-Abbas, R., & Al Hashemi, B. (2011). Luxury buying in the United Arab Emirates. *Journal of Business and Behavioural Sciences, 23*(3), 145–160.

Vupputuri, S., Hajat, C., Al-Houqani, M., Osman, O., Sreedharan, J., Ali, R., & Weitzman, M. (2016). Midwakh/dokha tobacco use in the Middle East: Much to learn. *Tobacco Control, 25*, 236–241. doi:10.1136/tobaccocontrol-2013-051530

Webster, N. (2016, September 2). UAE needs to address increasing cost of asthma. *The National.* Retrieved from https://www.thenational.ae/uae

Weqaya sample of 112, 301 UAE nationals in the Emirate screen in 2008–2009. (2008). Abu Dhabi: UAE University and Health Statistics Analysis, Health Authority Abu Dhabi.

World Culture Encyclopedia. (2017). Culture of UAE. Retrieved from http://www.everyculture.com/To-Z/United-Arab-Emirates.html

World Health Organization. (2000). *Global burden of disease, version 3*. Geneva, Switzerland: Author.

World Health Organization. (2013). Global action plan for the prevention and control of non-communicable disease 2013–2020. Retrieved from http://apps.who.int/iris/bitstream/10665/94384/1/9789241506236_eng.pdf?ua=1

World Health Organization. (2017). Noncommunicable diseases and their risk factors. Retrieved from http://www.who.int/ncds/introduction/en

Infection Control in Sierra Leone: A Global Issue

Elizabeth Holguin

The terms *international health* and *global health* are often used interchangeably. However, international health commonly refers to healthcare issues within the developing world, or low- to middle-income countries (LMICs). Global health refers to issues that go beyond individual country borders and require an interconnectedness of systems, disciplines, and policies. We have seen, through recent outbreaks such as severe acute respiratory syndrome (SARS), swine flu (H1N1), West Nile virus, and Ebola that the global community can be quickly affected. Resources must be shared and collaboration is essential to quickly stop the spread and adverse sequelae of these diseases. As in Ebola, outbreaks often stem from under-resourced areas that do not have the capacity to face the issue alone. It is essential to build a global community of cooperation, alliances, and partnerships to not only respond after the fact but to proactively prevent such breakdowns in public health infrastructure from occurring in the first place.

This chapter provides an overview of the country of Sierra Leone, my own experience attempting to implement an infection control program in a government hospital located in a Lassa fever–endemic region, and outlines several issues and challenges faced that are applicable to not only Sierra Leone but to any LMIC as well as underdeveloped and under-resourced areas within the United States.

OVERVIEW OF SIERRA LEONE

Sierra Leone is a country in West Africa with a population of approximately 6,018,888 (Central Intelligence Agency [CIA], 2017a). English is the official language but is used only by a literate minority. Mende is spoken mainly in the south and Temne is spoken mainly in the north. Krio, which is an English-based Creole first spoken by descendants of freed Jamaican slaves who were settled in the Freetown area, is the first language of about 10% of the population but is widely understood and used throughout the country (CIA, 2017a). The predominant religion is Islam (60%). Ten percent of the population practice Christianity while 30% practice other indigenous religions (CIA, 2017a).

Sierra Leone is a very youthful country; approximately 60% of the population is under the age of 25. Sierra Leone has a very high total fertility rate of almost five children per woman. There has been little decline due to a desire for large families, low levels of contraceptive use, and an early start to childbearing. However, Sierra Leone's population is mitigated by some of the world's highest infant, child, and maternal mortality rates, poverty, lack of clean drinking water and sanitation, poor nutrition, limited access to quality healthcare services, female genital cutting/mutilation (CIA, 2017b), poor feeding and hygienic practices, and overcrowded housing (World Health Organization [WHO], 2014a). High unemployment rates were one of the major causes of the civil war that took place from 1991 to 2002 and unemployment is a current threat to stability (CIA, 2017b). The unemployment rate is particularly high among youth and is attributed to high levels of illiteracy and unskilled labor, a lack of private sector jobs, and low pay (CIA, 2017a).

GOVERNMENTAL AND ADMINISTRATION STRUCTURE

Sierra Leone's governmental structure is similar to that of the United States in that it is divided into judicial, legislative, and executive branches. Sierra Leone is divided into Northern, Southern, and Eastern Regions, and the Western Area. The Western Area is divided between Western Rural and Western Urban, where the capital city, Freetown, is located; the majority of federal entities are located in Freetown. Each region is divided into 12 districts, which are further divided into chiefdoms, which are then subdivided into sections. Each district has a council that is comprised of district chair people, administrators, and counselors. Each chiefdom is governed by locally elected paramount chiefs. In 2004, the country divided into 19 local councils that are subdivided by 392 wards led by elected counselors due to recent decentralization efforts (WHO, 2014a). Sierra Leone has had extreme damage to its infrastructure due to an 11-year civil war that ended in 2002. In particular, major setbacks are still seen today in the health and development sectors (Scott, McMahon, Yumkella, Diaz, & George, 2014).

HEALTH ACCESS

Sierra Leone is almost last on the Human Development Report: 179 of 187 countries (United Nations Development Programme [UNDP], 2016). Due to poverty and lack of infrastructure, healthcare is fragmented. Health services in Sierra Leone are available through a network of health facilities. There are a total of 1,040 peripheral health units that include 40 hospitals (23 of which are government owned), community health centers, community health posts, and maternal and child health posts (WHO, 2014c). Besides contending with high costs to travel to and/or long distances to preferred healthcare facilities (Fleming et al., 2016), people needing healthcare in Sierra Leone lack treatment of surgical conditions and an adequate supply of anesthesia (Harris et al., 2015), childhood immunizations and adequate care for sick children (Scott et al., 2014), prenatal care (WHO, 2014c), and access to services for the disabled (Trani et al., 2011).

DISEASE BURDEN

Although noncommunicable diseases are on the rise with hypertension, diabetes, and mental illnesses increasing due to lifestyle changes and drug abuse (WHO, 2014a), the majority of illnesses and deaths are preventable in Sierra Leone. Most deaths can be attributed to nutritional deficiencies, pneumonia, diarrheal diseases, anemia, malaria, tuberculosis (TB), HIV/AIDS (WHO, 2014a), and helminth infections (Pullan, Smith, Jasrasaria, & Brooker, 2014). Malaria remains the most common cause of illness and death and accounts for about half of outpatient visits, 38% of hospital admissions, and 41% of hospital deaths among children under 5 years (WHO, 2014c). The citizens of Sierra Leone, as well as nearby countries like Guinea and Liberia, must also contend with viral hemorrhagic fevers such as Lassa and Ebola.

VIRAL HEMORRHAGIC FEVERS

Viral hemorrhagic fever is a term used to describe a syndrome that includes "fever, a constellation of initially nonspecific signs and symptoms, and a propensity for bleeding and shock" (Blumberg, Enria, & Bausch, 2014, p. 1). There are over 30 viruses that may cause viral hemorrhagic fever from four taxonomic families: Filoviridae, Arenaviridae, Bunyaviridae, and Flaviviridae (Blumberg et al., 2014). Almost all are zoonoses, with the exception of dengue hemorrhagic fever, and are usually named after the geographic region in which the first identified case originated (Blumberg et al., 2014). Little data exist on the exact mode of transmission from mammals to humans, but infection is presumed to occur from contact with the host's "virus-contaminated excreta," via mucous membrane or broken skin (Blumberg et al., 2014, p. 174). Human-to-human transmission occurs with many hemorrhagic fever viruses through direct contact with contaminated blood or other bodily fluids; this most often occurs through oral or mucous membrane exposure while providing care to sick family members or hospitalized patients or during funeral rituals that often involve touching the corpse prior to burial (Blumberg et al., 2014). Widespread outbreaks in an area are almost always the result of a high volume of cases in a particular healthcare setting in which basic infection control measures are no longer possible due to poverty or civil/political unrest (Blumberg et al., 2014) and the resulting lack of gloves and other personal protective equipment (PPE) and the reuse of unsterilized equipment such as needles (Bausch & Rollin, 2004).

LASSA FEVER

Most viral hemorrhagic fevers are only recognized when widespread outbreaks occur. However, Lassa fever, an Arenavirus, is endemic in West Africa and accounts for tens of thousands of cases annually (Richmond & Baglole, 2003; Shaffer et al., 2014). The Lassa virus is spread through contact with *Mastomys natalensis*, the "multimammate rat" (Centers for Disease Control and Prevention [CDC], 2014). The infected rodent is able to excrete the virus through its urine for a very long time, possibly its entire life (CDC, 2014). This particular species breeds frequently and produces large numbers of offspring (CDC, 2014).

Transmission to humans occurs because the rodents tend to enter homes, attracted to food that is not stored properly. There have also been some cases of certain populations consuming the rodents because they are used as a food source (CDC, 2014). Transmission can occur through ingestion or inhalation of the Lassa virus (CDC, 2014). The virus is shed in the urine and excrement. If humans come in direct contact with these by unknowingly touching soiled objects, eating contaminated food, or by exposure from open wounds, they may become infected (CDC, 2014).

Person-to-person transmission also may occur due to contact with an infected person's blood, tissue, secretions, or excretions; in addition, nosocomial transmission sometimes occurs when PPE is lacking or when needles are reused and not sterilized properly (CDC, 2014). After a 5- to 16-day incubation period, patients may present with a fever and many nonspecific symptoms that may include headache, sore throat, myalgia, abdominal pain, and diarrhea (Bausch et al., 2001; McCormick & Fisher-Hoch, 2002; Monath, Maher, Casals, Kissling, Cacciapuoti, 1974; Shaffer et al., 2014). More specific symptoms include conjunctival erythema, retrosternal pain, and facial swelling (Shaffer et al., 2014). In less than one-third of cases, mucosal and gastrointestinal bleeding occur (Shaffer et al., 2014). Death results from diminished effective circulating volume, shock, and multi-organ system failure (Peters, Lin, Anderson, Morrill, & Jahrling, 1989; Shaffer et al., 2014). Prompt early diagnosis is essential; there is no approved Lassa fever vaccine but the antiviral drug ribavirin can be effective if given within the first 6 days of the disease course (McCormick et al., 1986; Shaffer et al., 2014). Because diagnosis of Lassa and other highly communicable diseases can be delayed, it is essential to have a proper infection control program in place.

INFECTION CONTROL PROGRAM COMPONENTS

An infection control program has several essential components. The World Health Organization (WHO) has put forth several necessary elements that include prevention of transmission through standard and additional precautions; education and training of healthcare workers; protection of healthcare workers; identification of hazards and minimizing risks; routine practices such as aseptic technique, single use devices, instrument and equipment cleaning and sterilization, antibiotic usage, management of body fluid exposure, handling and use of blood and blood products, and responsible management of medical waste; effective work practices and procedures; surveillance; incident monitoring; outbreak investigation; infection control in specific situations; and research (WHO, 2004).

TRANSMISSION PREVENTION

Standard Precautions

For infection control, we focus on standard precautions that should be followed for every patient at all times, and additional transmission-based precautions that are case or disease specific, such as for contact, airborne, or droplet transmission. Standard precautions include (a) proper hand hygiene; (b) use of PPE when in contact with blood or bodily secretions; (c) handling patient care equipment or soiled linen in an appropriate manner; (d) prevention of accidental needle stick injuries or sharps injury; (e) environmental cleaning, usually with a bleach solution; (f) education on respiratory hygiene, or "cough etiquette" for patients and guests; (g) safe injection practices; and (h) appropriate handling of waste (Borlaug, 2016; WHO, 2004).

Airborne Precautions

Airborne precautions help to reduce airborne transmission when "droplet nuclei" or evaporated droplets are released and spread through the air, which may remain suspended in the air for long periods of time (WHO, 2004, p. 16). TB, measles, varicella, and SARS are spread through airborne transmission (Borlaug, 2016; WHO, 2004). For these patients, in addition to standard precautions, they must be placed in a negative airflow pressure room with the door closed at all times, an N 95 particulate respirator mask is required for anyone who has patient contact, and movement and transport of the patient should be limited (WHO, 2004).

Droplet Precautions

Droplet transmission can happen when large particle droplets generated from the infected person (coughing, sneezing, talking, or during procedures such as tracheal suctioning) come in contact with mucous membranes of the nose, mouth, or conjunctivae of a susceptible person (WHO, 2004). In addition to standard precautions, droplet precautions consist of placing the patient in a single room or in a room with a patient who is infected with the same pathogen, wearing a surgical mask when in close proximity to the patient, and placing a surgical mask on the patient during transport (WHO, 2004). Pneumonias, pertussis, diphtheria, influenza, mumps, meningitis (WHO, 2004), and smallpox (Borlaug, 2016) are spread through droplet transmission.

Contact Precautions

Contact precautions help to prevent diseases that are transmitted through direct or indirect contact with an infected person. Such diseases are norovirus, rotavirus, head lice (Borlaug, 2016), multiple antibiotic-resistant organisms, and skin infections (WHO, 2004). In addition to standard precautions, patients should be placed alone or with another patient with the same pathogen, anyone having patient contact should put on gloves and a clean nonsterile gown when entering the room, and patient transport should be limited (WHO, 2004). In addition, all reusable items should be cleaned and disinfected before removing from the patient's room and disposable items should be disposed of before leaving the room (Borlaug, 2016).

INFECTION CONTROL PROGRAM IMPLEMENTATION

The prior section provided a discussion of infection control program implementation in ideal conditions with easily accessible resources. This section outlines infection control program implementation in a very different context.

Upon arrival at Kenema Government Hospital (KGH), my first step was to spend several days observing routine patient care and hospital procedures. I spent time in an outpatient clinic, the nursing wards (both adult and pediatric patients), the TB ward, the Lassa fever ward, and the operating room. In the outpatient setting, a temporary structure similar to a mobile home, ECG electrodes were used repeatedly from patient to patient, so much so that they barely stuck to skin anymore. Electricity was unreliable, a problem everywhere but especially notable in the operating room. Nurses needed to have manual suctioning devices on hand. Many women were scheduled for cesarean sections because their labor had not progressed in their homes. For many, the intervention was too late for their infants. Chickens, cats, and dogs ran freely through the wards from time to time due to inadequately secured entry points. Window screens had gaping holes. To protect from malaria, each bed had a mosquito net, but some nets had holes in them as well. Most of the mattresses were visibly stained or soiled. Patients brought linens from home and families mainly supplied food. Scraps of soap bars were available for handwashing next to overused hand towels. No gloves were available in the wards unless the nurses purchased them themselves.

The TB ward was separated by male and female. The women were placed in a standard ward, in close proximity to nursing staff. The men, however, were located in a barn-like structure that was over 100 degrees inside. Some had beds and some laid only on scraps of cardboard on the floor. The Lassa ward did provide proper isolation for patients and medical staff did have access to PPE. However, there was inadequate capacity for housing a large number of patients and the amount of PPE was finite.

I spoke with administrators, physicians, and nurses to ascertain the issues that they face on a daily basis. I then identified one of the more senior nurses as the infection control nurse. I worked with him to identify further issues and to discuss next steps. The infection control nurse and I collaborated on a daily basis to identify the proper mode of training necessary for existing staff, as well as procedures for training of new staff. In addition, we aimed to create training refresher courses and brief competency exams for staff to complete at regular intervals.

IDENTIFIED ISSUES AND CHALLENGES

NURSING EDUCATION/LICENSING

Many of the nurses employed at KGH did not have proper education or training. It is very difficult to provide additional training for staff who are not sufficiently trained or familiar with the basics of nursing care. Lack of basic infection control prevention and PPE use training is widespread (Pathmanathan et al., 2014). Staff cannot be expected to be motivated to learn extra material when they are not paid on a regular basis; in fact, many were volunteering their time. Currently, there are 13 accredited nursing and midwifery training institutions in the country ("Sierra Leone News," 2016).

There is a major issue with illegal, unaccredited nursing and midwifery schools throughout Sierra Leone. These schools will accept those who do not have the required competencies to enter an accredited institution. This, in turn, produces certified nurses who are poorly prepared to practice clinically, which negatively impacts the professional standards of nursing ("Sierra Leone News," 2016). Youth in rural areas are susceptible to these types of institutions due to lack of accredited opportunities; of the 13 accredited institutions, only one is located in the eastern portion of Sierra Leone, with five in the west near the capital city of Freetown ("Sierra Leone News," 2016). Due to finances and logistics, many nursing students are forced to turn to less credible, illegal options for training to gain employment.

HUMAN RESOURCES FOR HEALTH

With the inception of the sustainable development goals (SDGs), the healthcare workforce has become a salient issue. It is a multifaceted issue, especially in LMICs. There are over four million people without access to quality healthcare services, largely related to a major shortage of workers, workers with mismatched or inadequate skill sets, and an uneven geographic distribution of health workers (WHO, 2017). Sierra Leone, similar to most African countries, has fewer than 20 physicians and fewer than 20 nurses or midwives per 10,000 people (WHO, 2010). By comparison, the United States has 50 to 99 nurses/midwives and 20 to 29 physicians per 10,000 people, while Canada and Australia have over 100 nurses and 20 to 29 physicians per 10,000 people (WHO, 2010).

Another major issue affecting patient care pertains to a phenomenon known as "brain drain." It refers to the emigration of highly talented professionals, like nurses, doctors, scientists, and professors, usually from LMICs to countries such as the United States, Canada, England, and Australia, thus leaving their countries of origin with a paucity of trained professionals. These professionals are usually attracted to a better quality of life and additional educational opportunities. This emigration can be especially detrimental to population health in countries that were under-resourced to begin with.

During the recent Ebola outbreak, it was noted through a surveillance effort that none of the surveyed districts had dedicated infection control supervisors to coordinate infection prevention and control procedures or quality assurance measures; those available within hospitals and holding centers were not likely to be competent in infection control practices (Pathmanathan et al., 2014). There were inadequate supplies of PPE as well as improper usage by staff (Pathmanathan et al., 2014). In general, there were notable widespread shortages of running water, incinerators to burn hazardous waste, chlorine, and blood collection supplies (Pathmanathan et al., 2014).

SUPPLIES AND FUNDING

The sheer lack of supplies was a major barrier when attempting to implement an infection control program in KGH. How could infection control measures be enforced when there are no gloves or soap, let alone gowns, masks, proper facilities, etc.? I was not in Sierra Leone long enough to determine funding issues, but from staff report, corruption may have been a factor.

Policies are needed to ensure proper funding pathways from the Ministry of Health down to each hospital or clinic so that patients can be cared for in the proper manner and rest assure that they are receiving care in a safe environment. In addition, healthcare workers should not have to risk their lives to come to work each day. Hundreds of nurses and physicians lost their lives in the recent Ebola outbreak. The WHO attributes high infection rates to shortages of PPE, improper use of PPE, inadequate staffing to cover the needs of such a large outbreak, and compassion driving staff to work in isolation wards beyond the number of hours considered to be safe (WHO, 2014b).

POLICY IMPLICATIONS

It is essential for nurses to obtain health or public policy positions in national or international organizations to influence decision making at the highest levels. As nurses, it is important to go beyond the "nursing bubble" (Shamian, 2014) to influence factors in other health, social, and economic domains. Nurses understand the needs of their patients and communities. Nursing is the largest healthcare profession, with the "potential to be a leading powerhouse for positive change and innovation" (Holguin, Hughes, & Shamian, 2017, p. 201), and can play a critical role in impacting the social determinants of health for their patient populations (Holguin et al., 2017). By acquiring leadership roles in government or national organizations, nurses can ensure that the multifaceted issues that patients face will be brought to the forefront of healthcare and social policy decision making. As a global community, nurses in the developed world cannot allow fellow nurses in developing countries to continue to work in conditions that are life-threatening, or tolerate patients facing unnecessary and preventable threats to their well-being and livelihood on a daily basis while their basic human needs are not met. Nurses have the power and ability to influence nursing education and regulation;

hospital and healthcare system policies, strategies, and guidelines; social determinants of health for patients; and governmental or institutional financial resource allocation.

SUMMARY

Nurses are in a unique position to assist in designing an improved healthcare system that can lead to universal health coverage because they understand the intricacies of patients' needs as well as the inner workings of the healthcare system. Nurses must secure a seat at the policy table for real and significant change to occur. To begin making changes in your current position, you can join your own institution's infection control committee, a shared governance committee, hospital board, or local public health organization or board. It is important to join national and international nursing organizations to form professional relationships and support networks. Doing so will allow you to learn from other nurses and unite as a global community, making nursing a stronger and more effective profession.

REFERENCES

Bausch, D. G., Demby, A. H., Coulibaly, M., Kanu, J., Goba, A., Bah, A., . . . Rollin, P. (2001). Lassa fever in Guinea: I. Epidemiology of human disease and clinical observations. *Vector Borne and Zoonotic Diseases, 1*(4), 269–281. doi:10.1089/15303660160025903

Bausch, D. G., & Rollin, P. E. (2004). Responding to epidemics of Ebola hemorrhagic fever: Progress and lessons learned from recent outbreaks in Uganda, Gabon, and Congo. In W. M. Scheld, B. E. Murray, & J. M. Hughes (Eds.), *Emerging Infections 6*. Washington, DC: ASM Press.

Blumberg, L., Enria, D., & Bausch, D. G. (2014). Viral haemorrhagic fevers. In J. Farrar, P. J. Hotez, T. Junghanss, G. Kang, D. Lalloo, & N. White (Eds.), *Manson's tropical diseases* (23rd ed.). China: Elsevier Saunders.

Borlaug, G. (2016). *Infection control and prevention – Standard precautions: Infection control principles and practices for local health agencies.* Madison, WI: Wisconsin Department of Health Services. Retrieved from https://www .dhs.wisconsin.gov/ic/precautions.htm

Centers for Disease Control and Prevention. (2014). Lassa fever: Transmission. Retrieved from https://www.cdc.gov/vhf/lassa/transmission/index.html

Central Intelligence Agency. (2017). *The World Factbook: Sierra Leone.* Washington, DC: Author. Retrieved from https://www.cia.gov/library/publications/the-world-factbook/geos/sl.html

Central Intelligence Agency. (2017). *The World Factbook: United States.* Washington, DC: Author. Retrieved from https://www.cia.gov/library/publications/the-world-factbook/geos/us.html

Fleming, L. C., Ansumana, R., Bockarie, A. S., Alejandre, J. D., Owen, K. K., Bangura, U., ... Jacobsen, K. H. (2016). Health-care availability, preference, and distance for women in urban Bo, Sierra Leone. *International Journal of Public Health, 61,* 1079–1088. doi:10.1007/s00038-016-0815-y

Harris, M. J., Kamara, T. B., Hanciles, E., Newberry, C., Junkins, S. R., & Pace, N. L. (2015). Accessing unmet anaesthesia need in Sierra Leone: A secondary analysis of a cluster-randomized, cross-sectional, countrywide survey. *African Health Sciences, 15*(3), 1028–1033. doi:10.4314/ahs.v15i3.43

Holguin, E., Hughes, F., & Shamian, J. (2017). Transnational nursing organizations paving the way for global health: The International Council of Nurses as exemplar. In W. Rosa (Ed.), *A new era in global health: Nursing and the United Nations 2030 agenda for sustainable development* (pp. 201–221). New York, NY: Springer Publishing.

McCormick, J. B., & Fisher-Hoch, S. P. (2002). Lassa fever. *Current Topics in Microbiology and Immunology, 262,* 75–109. doi:10.1007/978-3-642-56029-3_4

McCormick, J. B., King, I. J., Webb, P. A., Scribner, C. L., Craven, R. B., Johnson, K. M., ... Belmont-Williams, R. (1986). Lassa fever: Effective therapy with ribavirin. *The New England Journal of Medicine, 314*(1), 20–26. doi:10.1056/NEJM198601023140104

Monath, T. P., Maher, M., Casals, J., Kissling, R. E., & Cacciapuoti, A. (1974). Lassa fever in the Eastern Province of Sierra Leone, 1970–1972. II. Clinical observations and virological studies on selected hospital cases. *The American Journal of Tropical Medicine and Hygiene, 23,* 1140–1149. doi:10.4269/ajtmh.1974.23.1140

Pathmanathan, I., O'Connor, K. A., Adams, M. L., Rao, C. Y., Kilmarx, P. H., ... Clarke, K. R. (2014). Rapid assessment of Ebola infection prevention and control needs—Six districts, Sierra Leone, October 2014. *Morbidity and Mortality Weekly Report, 63*(49), 1172–1174.

Peters, C. J., Lin, C.-T., Anderson, G. W., Morrill, J. C., & Jahrling, P. B. (1989). Pathogenesis of viral hemorrhagic fevers: Rift Valley fever and Lassa fever contrasted. *Reviews of Infectious Diseases, 11*(Suppl. 4), S743–S749. doi:10.1093/clinids/11.Supplement_4.S743

Pullan, R. L., Smith, J. L., Jasrasaria, R., & Brooker, S. J. (2014). Global numbers of infection and disease burden of soil transmitted helminth infections in 2010. *Parasites and Vectors, 7*(37), 1–19. doi:10.1186/1756-3305-7-37.

Richmond, J. K., & Baglole, D. J. (2003). Lassa fever: Epidemiology, clinical features, and social consequences. *British Medical Journal, 327*, 1271–1275. doi:10.1136/bmj.327.7426.1271

Scott, K., McMahon, S., Yumkella, F., Diaz, T., & George, A. (2014). Navigating multiple options and social relationships in plural health systems: A qualitative study exploring healthcare seeking for sick children in Sierra Leone. *Health Policy and Planning, 29*(3), 292–301. doi:10.1093/heapol/czt016

Shaffer, J. G., Grant, D. S., Schieffelin, J. S., Boisen, M. L., Goba, A., Hartnett, J. N., ... Garry, R. F. (2014). Lassa fever in post-conflict Sierra Leone. *PLoS Neglected Tropical Diseases, 8*(3), e2748. doi:10.1371/journal.pntd.0002748

Shamian, J. (2014). Global perspectives on nursing and its contribution to health-care and health policy: Thoughts on an emerging policy model. *Canadian Journal of Nursing Leadership, 27*(4), 44–50. doi:10.12927/cjnl.2015.24140

Sierra Leone News: Unaccredited nursing schools are unacceptable – Health Ministry. (2016, April 14). Awoko Newspaper. Retrieved from http://awoko.org/2016/04/14/sierra-leone-news-unaccredited-nursing-schools-are-unacceptable-health-ministry

Trani, J., Browne, J., Kett, M., Bah, O., Morlai, T., Bailey, N., & Groce, N. (2011). Access to health care, reproductive health and disability: A large-scale survey in Sierra Leone. *Social Science and Medicine, 73*(10), 1477–1489. doi:10.1016/j.socscimed.2011.08.040

United Nations Development Programme. (2016). Human Development Reports. Retrieved from http://hdr.undp.org/en/countries

World Health Organization. (2004). *Practical guidelines for infection control in health care facilities.* SEARO Regional Publication No. 41, WPRO Regional Publication, India: Author. Retrieved from http://www.wpro.who.int/publications/docs/practical_guidelines_infection_control.pdf

World Health Organization. (2010). *World health statistics 2010.* Geneva, Switzerland: Author. https://books.google.com/books?hl=en&lr=&id=Z69vxfRfFIsC&oi=fnd&pg=PA1&dq=health+workforce+distribution+sierra+leone&ots=cGRKfhIFby&sig=0dvvIjy6ii5whdfuILA_phEg0mE#v=onepage&q&f=false

World Health Organization. (2014a). *Sierra Leone: Introduction to country context.* African Health Observatory. Retrieved from http://www.aho.afro.who.int/ profiles_information/index.php/Sierra_Leone:Introduction_to_Country_Context

World Health Organization. (2014b). Unprecedented number of medical staff infected with Ebola. Retrieved from www.who.int/mediacentre/news/ ebola/25-august-2014/en

World Health Organization. (2014c). *The health system.* African Health Observatory. Retrieved from http://www.aho.afro.who.int/profiles_information/index .php/Sierra_Leone:The_Health_System

World Health Organization. (2017). Health workforce: Education and training. Retrieved from http://www.who.int/hrh/education/en

HIV and Male Circumcision in Swaziland

R. Kevin Mallinson
Bongani T. Sibandze

The age of global nursing is on us. More than any other time in history, the impact of health policies is transnational; increasingly, one country's health initiative affects the health and well-being of the neighboring countries. Health outcomes are influenced by a myriad of factors including poverty, fluctuations in economics, or changes in climate patterns. Traditionally, health policies have been developed by politicians, physicians, and public health experts; however, when few individuals make decisions that affect millions of persons, there may be a limited understanding of the challenges and dangers of rolling out a health initiative in a specific culture, country, or region. Nurses must engage as equal partners in the development, implementation, and evaluation of global health policies.

In most parts of the world, and Africa in particular, nurses are delivering the majority of the health services and are stakeholders in any policies affecting healthcare. It is imperative that the design and implementation of health policies integrate the perspectives of professional nurses. Nursing's inherent values would ensure that social justice, cultural respect, and effective cross-cultural communication contribute to the design of effective health policies. Successful global health policies will maximize benefits to many without causing undue harm to vulnerable populations. Poorly planned health policies may be ineffective and costly. Without careful consideration of its implications, a poorly designed health program can be counterproductive.

Africa has been severely affected by the human immunodeficiency virus (HIV) pandemic for nearly 50 years. The sub-Saharan region of the continent shoulders three quarters of the global disease burden and, yet, has only 3% of the world's healthcare workers. The morbidity and mortality associated with the HIV pandemic has affected more than individuals and their families—communities have been decimated, economies have been weakened, and political stability has been threatened. In addition to the evidence-based interventions to control the spread of the HIV virus (e.g., safer sex initiatives, treatment with antiretrovirals), African leaders have been anxious to integrate innovative, effective approaches to HIV prevention. However, the introduction of new biomedical interventions should be carefully considered by a diverse team of social scientists and healthcare professionals, including professional nurses.

A case example is presented to outline the complexities of implementing an "American" health initiative across an African country. The case highlights the unintended consequences for a vulnerable society when a global health policy is designed with limited regard for the customs, practices, and resources of the country. Recommendations for effectively engaging nurses in the development, implementation, and evaluation of global health policies are offered.

CASE EXAMPLE: VOLUNTARY MALE MEDICAL CIRCUMCISION IN SWAZILAND

An estimated 4,000 new HIV infections occur in the sub-Saharan region of Africa each day (Kharsany & Karim, 2016). The country with the highest seroprevalence of HIV infection—27% of the adult population—is the Kingdom of Swaziland (World Health Organization, 2013). The country's small population of 1.5 million people is strikingly homogeneous; approximately 97% of the people are members of the Swazi tribe. Over the five decades of the HIV pandemic, the Swazi people, and their healthcare workers in particular, have experienced unprecedented levels of morbidity and mortality. The life expectancy at birth for a Swazi infant in 2006 was 42 years. As the result of antiretroviral medications for HIV disease, the life expectancy for a Swazi male in 2015 was up to 57 years; for females, the life expectancy was at 61 years (World Health Organization, 2016, Statistics section, p. 1).

The majority of new HIV infections among adolescents and adults in Swaziland are the result of unprotected vaginal intercourse between heterosexual partners. There are several drivers of the epidemic; in addition to poverty, there are cultural customs that frustrate HIV prevention efforts. Swaziland has a polygynous society; a man can have more than one wife at the same time. Although generally frowned upon by the society, it is not uncommon for a married man to have girlfriends as well. A major risk factor for acquiring—and spreading—HIV infection is having multiple partners. Although more women become infected with HIV, more men die from HIV-related causes. Men may be less likely to attend clinics, receive a diagnosis, and engage in treatment (McNeish, 2016).

EMERGENCY RESPONSE

Understandably, scientists globally have sought interventions that would significantly reduce the impact of HIV infections. At the International AIDS Society conference in Montreal in 2006, a [Caucasian] physician from the United States presented the findings of a second major randomized clinical trial of medical male circumcision in Africa. The study provided mounting evidence that male circumcision could significantly reduce a man's chances of acquiring HIV infection through vaginal sex. The presenter concluded with a recommendation that a male medical circumcision initiative be immediately rolled out across sub-Saharan Africa to reduce new infections in men. A nurse in that presentation pondered, "Doesn't it seem a bit like colonial paternalism for a White American physician to advocate for cutting the foreskin of a Black African man's penis *for his own good*?"

In response to the research findings presented in Montreal, the United States' President's Emergency Plan for AIDS Relief (PEPFAR) team—in collaboration with UNAIDS—developed an ambitious initiative to promote voluntary medical male circumcision in sub-Saharan countries with high incidence rates of new HIV infections. In 2009, a voluntary medical male circumcision program, termed the Accelerated Saturation Initiative (ASI), was adopted in the Kingdom of Swaziland. At the time, a mere 8% of Swazi males were circumcised (Central Statistics Office, 2017, p. 176). Being a small country, it was envisioned that the program would quickly achieve its target to circumcise 80% of the adolescent and adult males between the ages of 15 and 49 years; then, Swaziland would serve as a model for other countries to follow. History, however, will record that the efforts to circumcise the adolescent and adult males in Swaziland proved much more difficult than predicted.

DISMAL CIRCUMCISION OUTCOMES

The ASI circumcision initiative in Swaziland began with educational messaging for the public, healthcare worker sensitization, and promotion by well-known celebrities. In 2011, the Swazi monarch, King Mswati III, spoke in support, encouraging the males of the country to be circumcised. Physicians, nurse midwives, and nurses were trained to perform the procedure. Throughout the country, one frequently encountered signs, pamphlets, and billboards with the program slogan *Soka Uncobe* (siSwati for *cut and conquer*) under the image of a cartoon male figure with a muscular physique who is holding his arms up as if claiming victory over the enemy (i.e., HIV). Over the years of the campaign, a tacit implication was promoted through the campaign that "any Swazi male who cares about those he loves will be circumcised." As a result of this erroneous message, many healthcare providers assumed an insidious mindset that a male who chose not to be circumcised was ignorant, ill-informed, or untrustworthy. In spite of a well-funded campaign and questionable recruitment tactics, very few Swazi males have chosen to be circumcised.

After a couple of years, the ASI voluntary medical male circumcision (VMMC) program in Swaziland had reached less than 20% of its initial goal; a yearlong intensive campaign in 2011, costing more than $15 million of PEPFAR funding, failed to significantly improve the dismal numbers. As of 2014, it was estimated that only 24% of Swazi adolescent and adult males had been circumcised (Fitzgerald et al., 2016). Similar VMMC programs in neighboring countries also failed to meet their program targets. The KwaZulu-Natal province of neighboring South Africa reported meeting only 22% to 38% of its VMMC program targets in its numerous locations (Smith, 2012). Similarly, Moyo, Mhloyi, Chevo, and Rusinga (2015) reported that nearby Zimbabwe had barely met 10% of its targeted number of male circumcisions with its VMMC initiative.

EARLY INFANT MALE CIRCUMCISION

A separate, though related, program to circumcise infant males was launched in 2010 to provide Swaziland with long-term sustainability of this approach to HIV prevention. The Early Infant Male Circumcision (EIMC) program was able to perform more than 5,000 EIMCs in its first 5 years of operation (Fitzgerald et al., 2016). An estimated 80% of the EIMCs were performed during the immediate postpartum period before discharge from the facility. There were no reported adverse effects for the infants. However, the program faced challenges that may have resulted from how the EIMC initiative was designed and implemented in the Swazi healthcare context.

As with the VMMC program for adolescents and adult males, the EIMC initiative had healthcare workforce implications. Fitzgerald et al. (2016) noted that there was a need to task-shift the major responsibility of the EIMCs to nursing personnel in the facility. This required additional training and mentorship, shifting personnel from their regular posts, and requiring "additional tasks without providing additional compensation" (p. S83).

There were additional challenges to the EIMC program that were unique. If the facility was to perform the circumcision of the infant before the mother and baby were discharged, the education had to be provided in the prenatal period and counseling for informed consent completed in a very short timeframe (Fitzgerald et al., 2016). Similar to the erroneous messages conveyed to adolescent and adult males in the VMMC program, mothers were presented with a coercive expectation that "any good mother would do this for her child." As Swazi men do not traditionally attend prenatal sessions or come to the hospital for the baby's birth, they often had limited—or no—ability to contribute to the decision to have their male child circumcised. In the absence of the baby's father, the pressure on mothers to quickly make the "right" decision is unethical. Circumcision involves removing a small part of the male anatomy. The male (i.e., father) is traditionally the head of the family and should have been included in the decision to circumcise. When the father learned that the procedure had already been performed on his son, it may have led to conflict in the parents' relationship.

LESSONS LEARNED FROM THE CIRCUMCISION INITIATIVES IN SWAZILAND

There is a preponderance of convincing evidence that VMMC effectively lowers a male's risk of acquiring HIV during vaginal sex, poses no undue risk, and does not affect function or reduce sexual satisfaction. So, why would men not elect to reduce their risk of acquiring HIV infection with an evidence-based intervention that results in very few complications or side effects? There are numerous personal, familial, social, and political reasons why the VMMC program in Swaziland failed to meet its expected outcomes. First, and foremost, is that VMMC is a surgical intervention; it is not as simple or innocuous as a vaccination. Even more so, a vaccination program is rolled out across a community because the vaccinated person acquires protection for self *and others*; VMMC only provides partial protection for the male who undergoes the procedure. Nurses have an appreciation for the lived experience of persons, the importance of gender roles and identities, and the resistance that can develop when persons are feeling coerced to do something that they may not want. If the knowledge and insights of professional nurses had been used to design and implement the circumcision program, it might have been more successful and less damaging to the Swazi people and the reputation of America.

PARTIAL PROTECTION

The research that led to the VMMC programs had demonstrated that males received a 60% reduction in the chance of acquiring HIV during vaginal intercourse after being circumcised. Circumcision is not 100% effective in protecting a male from acquiring HIV during vaginal intercourse. Gray et al. (2007), the authors of one of the leading randomized clinical trials of VMMC, warned that there "is a critical need to practice safer sex after circumcision" (p. 665). The concept of partial protection may have been a complex one to explain to males being recruited for VMMC in Swaziland. Healthcare providers are responsible for providing culturally appropriate and medically accurate information when describing the limited effectiveness of circumcision in preventing HIV infections (Milford et al., 2016). The VMMC counselors had to adequately respond to males who would ask questions such as "If one had to continue to use a condom for protection, what was the point of undergoing the circumcision procedure?"

The VMMC program was well funded and provided a new income opportunity for health-related nongovernmental organizations in Swaziland. Some organizations that were unwilling to recommend or provide condoms (due to their faith, mission, or funding sources) were benefitting from recruiting males for circumcision. The message to continue safer sex after circumcision would have been avoided in these settings.

THE "EMERGENCY" ROLLOUT

There is no doubt that the HIV pandemic was an emergency situation for the Swazi people. However, the rapid nature with which the ASI was rolled out across the country may have contributed to its failures. The rapid rollout of the VMMC initiative did not permit enough time for adequate consultation with local chiefs, traditional leaders, or others who may have been able to persuade uncircumcised men to consider this novel approach to HIV prevention. Similar programs in South Africa may have failed, in part, because of the inadequate training of health providers responsible for communicating complex information to males confused by the options (Milford et al., 2016).

The accelerated program may have led to some unintended consequences. The Swazi ASI program was designed to target the "most at-risk" adolescent and adult males for the prevention intervention. Therefore, men who were HIV seronegative were eligible to be circumcised; men who were already HIV infected were not going to receive any added protection by undergoing the procedure. The health providers noted that HIV-infected men were not eligible for VMMC. It became apparent that men who had been in the queue for counseling and testing and were turned away without being circumcised were likely to be HIV infected. As many circumcisions were performed in army "surgical tents" set up in open fields, the community was quick to notice who was not eligible and began rumors that stigmatized these men. The program had to adapt by circumcising HIV seropositive men if they presented for the procedure.

Kelly et al. (2013) asserted that "biomedical technologies are neither ethically nor morally neutral" (p. 181). The VMMC implementers, believing that they have the best intentions, may have diminished the legitimate concerns of the local consultants and accelerated a circumcision initiative because their public health training assured them that "they know what is best" to reduce new HIV infections. Consequently, the VMMC program was perceived by some Swazi professionals as a modern-day colonial imposition. The development of effective and lasting interventions to reduce HIV infections requires programs that are based on a preponderance of convincing evidence, patience in implementation, and adaptation to the cultural context.

MONETARY INCENTIVES

There was no cost to the male who wished to be circumcised. However, private physicians received a payment (~US$60) for each circumcision completed. Similarly, community health workers (CHWs) in local communities who recruited men for VMMC received a small, unspecified amount of local currency (emalangeni) for each eligible male who was persuaded to come in for the procedure. There are concerns that paying monetary incentives to the CHWs who recruited men for circumcision may have undermined complete disclosure; a CHW might have withheld crucial details to recruit as many males as possible for the procedure. In a country where 63% of the population is living below the poverty level, nursing personnel often worked the circumcision services during their vacation days to earn extra income.

NOT CONSIDERING THE CULTURE

In the Swazi culture, a man is a proud, responsible man. Traditionally, he should be the head of the family, a [proverbial] warrior, who is able to provide for his family's needs. McNeish (2016) noted that the high rates of unemployment left some Swazi men unable to feed their families. The inability to fulfill their culturally defined roles as "men" may contribute to ineffective coping such as violence or substance abuse. In a culture that does not have a history of traditional circumcision (e.g., as a custom of passage from boy to man), removing a Swazi man's foreskin may raise concerns about masculinity, strength, and the maintenance of one's male persona. Circumcision may be perceived by some as a form of emasculation and the procedure is, after all, permanent.

Kelly et al. (2012) found that cultural concerns about VMMC in Papua New Guinea focused around masculinity, attractiveness, and fertility following the procedure. Older Swazi men are particularly reluctant to have a part of their "manhood" surgically removed. Some of the VMMC literature assured males that females would find a circumcised male more sexually attractive or that the male's sexual performance could improve (in the face of no evidence to support either of these notions). The truth is that no one knew how female sexual partners would respond to males without foreskin.

Though rarely discussed openly with the visiting *umlungu* (White person), many Swazi people have fervent beliefs in witchcraft. There are unscrupulous traditional practitioners who are notorious in using human body parts to assure that their curses, spells, and incantations will be successful. Swazi males have expressed concerns that their excised foreskin could be sold to witchdoctors (IRIN, 2013; Smith, 2012), consequently putting them at risk for a host of unfortunate events. The fear of being "bewitched" is a powerful impediment to circumcision for Swazi males.

MESSAGING

Indeed, the VMMC campaign in Swaziland was an expensive, resource-laden effort to reduce new HIV infections in heterosexual males. However, there were also unintended outcomes of the VMMC campaign. The slogan for the campaign was *Soka Uncobe* (siSwati for *cut and conquer*). Smith (2012) found that some Swazi men interpreted the catchphrase to mean that once one was circumcised, one would not have to continue with other prevention methods such as using condoms or reducing multiple partners. Some men who were voluntarily circumcised mistakenly thought that they had "conquered" HIV and could safely engage in unprotected sex with their female partners. The hyperbole in the messaging may have undermined the vigilance among men who had accepted the VMMC intervention. After decades of needing to "condomize," Swazi men have grown weary of HIV messages that seem to blame them for the spreading epidemic (McNeish, 2016) and an intervention like circumcision that provided protection against HIV—albeit partial protection—was enticing.

The misinterpretation of the *Soka Uncobe* slogan may have put both men and women at risk for becoming infected. Some HIV seronegative men were circumcised and, subsequently, became infected by having unsafe vaginal intercourse. Unfortunately, this led to a common myth among Swazi men that Americans (purposely) infect a man when he undergoes the circumcision procedure. It is not the first time that Africans have questioned the motives of influential outsiders. A sarcastic quip shared among Swazi men is that the acronym AIDS stands for "American Ideas for Discouraging Sex."

EXERCISING POWER

Whenever there is a partnership between the United States and a less-developed country like Swaziland, there is a power differential that threatens the authentic decision making of those receiving the necessary funds. The VMMC rollout across Swaziland was rapid and involved large amounts of money to assure the necessary materials, messaging, and trained personnel willing to undertake the effort. Though the program was designed to have a minimal impact on the already overburdened healthcare system in the country, it was significantly disruptive to the medical facilities and nursing personnel who were responsible for delivering the VMMC services (Fitzgerald et al., 2016).

There were HIV experts who were not convinced that the VMMC program was the right option for Swaziland. Some noted that, in contrast to the prevailing scientific notions, the 2006 to 2007 demographic and health survey of Swazi homesteads (Central Statistics Office, 2007, p. 227) revealed that males who were circumcised had a higher prevalence of HIV infection (21.8%) than did men who were not circumcised (19.5%). This seemed to question the need for circumcision in the country. Some Swazi professionals felt that the health ministry acquiesced to the imposition of the initiative because of the promise of much-needed funding (IRIN, 2013); similarly, other HIV professionals felt pressured to agree to the "exercise in bullying" by the U.S. partners for fear of losing funding (Smith, 2012, Mixed Messages section, p. 1). On the health facility level, the pressure to meet the circumcision program target numbers may have unduly influenced personnel shifts and budgeting decisions that adversely affected other crucial health services.

ETHICAL NURSING PRACTICE AND MALE CIRCUMCISION

The International Council of Nurses (ICN) *Code of Ethics* (www.ich.ch/who-we-are/code-of-ethics-for-nurses) outlines the four core elements guiding ethical nursing practice. Each of the principles has relevance for nurses who could have contributed to the design and implementation of the VMMC initiative in Swaziland. The first principle of the code underscores that nurses must engage with persons, families, and communities in a manner that respects their human rights, values, customs, and spiritual beliefs. If the circumcision initiatives had founded their approach on this principle, there would have been an appropriate assessment of the potential impact of this innovative HIV prevention intervention in the Swazi context. Furthermore, the design would have been a collaboration between global partners and not a "one size fits all" approach that was too rushed to consider the local customs and concerns.

The code's second element requires that nurses hold themselves accountable for their interactions with clients. The nurse is responsible for having the requisite knowledge (e.g., about the complexities of circumcision and partial protection) and assures that new technologies are safe and maintain the dignity of clients. There is evidence that the rapid scale-up of the VMMC initiative may have led to providers being unprepared to address complicated questions posed by potential clients. Ethically, nurses must act in a manner that instills confidence in the profession.

Additional ethical expectations are noted in the third principle of the code. Specifically, nurses are obligated to challenge unethical practices and settings. The Swazi nurses observed how the VMMC and infant circumcision programs added undue burden to their workload and altered usual health service delivery. Nurses were aware of when circumcision "counseling" bordered on blatant coercion or patients' rights were being ignored. If the nurses had been educated, empowered, and mentored, these transgressions provided opportunities to act in an ethical manner.

The last of the four principles of the ICN *Code of Ethics* maintains that nurses have an ethical obligation to "safeguard" persons, families, and communities when the actions of others put them at risk. If nurses were engaged in the design of the VMMC initiative and determining the goals of the program, this principle could have guided decisions that ensured the rights of the males to be properly informed to make their own choices about circumcision. The workload issues for nursing personnel could have considered equity, safety, and appropriate compensation for extra work duties. This principle could also endorse an effective health provider training program that led to the recruiters, counselors, and practitioners feeling confident about their knowledge and skills in delivering the circumcision services to the clients.

ENGAGING NURSES IN HEALTH POLICY DECISIONS

Nurses may not believe that they have a legitimate seat at the table when health policies are developed. Upvall (2012) suggested that the perceived "powerlessness" in global nursing might be best addressed by assuming a feminist perspective, and basing programs on professional values of "social justice [and] critical reflection" (p. 58). Nurses in Africa have been noted for their inspiring ingenuity, innovation, and perseverance in the face of severe shortages of staff and resources (Mallinson & Sibandze, 2017). Indeed, nurses are skilled at "making do" when health policies leave them with no other choice. Rather than being reactive to the decisions of others, nurses need the skills to proactively engage in making health policy.

There are numerous nursing "capacity-building" programs in sub-Saharan Africa. Too often, the focus of an initiative is limited to clinical improvements, staff management, and increasing the efficiency of patient care services; there is much less emphasis placed on the development of the leadership skills nurses need to fully participate as stakeholders in health policy meetings. Rather than having the funded professor from the West (e.g., American) take the lead, capacity-building programs could provide opportunities for local nurse leaders to make formal presentations before influential stakeholders in their community or country. Nurses could be encouraged, mentored, and provided the technical assistance to prepare reports of ongoing projects, the findings of research studies, or updates on major health initiatives. An emphasis could be placed on how nursing's perspectives have contributed to the success of the programs, the community's satisfaction with the cultural adaptations, or the innovative approaches to care. Local nurses can be mentored in how to situate themselves on committees and boards that make health policy in their region.

It is important for nurses to have the academic credentials to support their place at the policy table. Nurses in Swaziland have extraordinarily few opportunities to access information that Western nurses take for granted; the unstable and slow Internet access makes it a challenge to obtain online articles and educational materials. Weaver (1998) strongly encouraged nurses in the international community to apply for educational grants (e.g., Fulbright Scholarships or Rockefeller Foundation funding), research funding (e.g., Fogarty International fellowships), or programmatic support (e.g., United Nations funding). Nurses who have the opportunity to study outside of their country may learn that they contribute significantly to interdisciplinary workgroups, develop assertiveness skills, explore ethical issues, and critically examine alternative philosophies. Such opportunities expand one's horizons and sharpen one's resolve to shape health services in their home country.

Nurses should also be encouraged to publish their work. The written word allows nurses to communicate their insights about the lived experience of clients, the subtle cultural aspects affecting a program's outcomes, or the social injustice that results from a poorly designed intervention. Nurses can learn how to inform, inspire, and influence others through rich and meaningful discourses. Through effective storytelling, nurses can provide ethical guidance and cultural adaptations that could ensure the successful implementation of a health policy.

Depending on the culture, nurses can be encouraged to seek elected or appointed positions in governmental health structures. If nurses served as the minister of health, a member of parliament, or in similar positions of power, they may have authentic input into the development and implementation of major health policies. Mentorship, guidance, and support for these nurses may come from the ICN or any of its member organizations (i.e., national nurse associations).

Engaging nurses in health policy dialogue also begins in the basic nursing program. Nursing students need to know that a professional responsibility is to apply their knowledge, insights, and professional values to policies that will promote and protect the health and well-being of all members of their society, particularly vulnerable persons and populations. The basic program can provide opportunities to debate contemporary health issues and demonstrate how each policy decision has its implications. Role modeling and role-play activities can be used to develop effective negotiating skills. Students could engage in interactive assignments that strengthen their emotional intelligence so that they are better able to empathize with others who have opposing views. Carefully adapting exercises and materials to align with the local culture will help avoid conflict and build the students' self-efficacy to advocate successfully.

SUMMARY

The unfolding complexities of globalization have led to global health policies being developed by politicians, physicians, and public health advocates as well as economists, pharmaceutical conglomerates, and members of civil society. The nurses are, most often, the end users in this process, responsible for delivering the health services to the population. The voice of nurses must be included in determining what should be done, how it should be done, and how protections for the society's most vulnerable members will be assured.

Nurses have based their professional practice on principles of social justice, respect for persons, and advocacy for the most vulnerable persons and populations. These basic values are the foundation on which health policy decisions can be built. In many countries, nurses are perceived as trustworthy professionals who are dedicated to the health and well-being of their communities. The development and implementation of successful global health policies will need to consider cultural influences, variations in human response, and the individual's right to choose. Nurses have a unique body of knowledge and deserve a legitimate seat at the policy table. The agenda, therefore, should include placing nurses in health policy arenas and providing the support and resources that they need to fully participate as valuable stakeholders.

REFERENCES

Central Statistics Office. (2007). Swaziland demographic and health survey 2006–07. Retrieved from http://microdata.worldbank.org/index.php/catalog/1492

Fitzgerald, L., Benzerga, W., Mirira, M., Adamu, T., Shissler, T., Bitchong, R., . . . Maziya, V. (2016). Scaling up early infant male circumcision: Lessons from the Kingdom of Swaziland. *Global Health: Science and Practice, 4*(1), S76–S86. doi:10.9745/GHSP-D-15-00186

Gray, R. H., Kigozi, G., Serwadda, D., Makumbi, F., Watya, S., Nalugoda, F., . . . Wawer, M. J. (2007). Male circumcision for HIV prevention in men in Rakai, Uganda: A randomized trial. *Lancet, 369*(9562), 657–666. doi:10.1016/S0140-6736(07)60313-4

IRIN. (2013). Circumcision plans go awry in Swaziland. *IRIN News.* Retrieved from http://www.irinnews.org/news/2013/05/13

Kelly, A., Kupul, M., Aeno, H., Shih, P., Naketrumb, R., Neo, J., . . . Vallely, A. (2013). Why women object to male circumcision to prevent HIV in a moderate-prevalence setting. *Qualitative Health Research, 23*(2), 180–193. doi:10.1177/1049732312467234

Kelly, A., Kupul, M., Naketrumb, R., Aeno, H., Neo, J., Fitzgerald, L., . . . Vallely, A. (2012). More than just a cut: A qualitative study of penile practices and their relationship to masculinity, sexuality, and contagion and their implications for HIV prevention in Papua, New Guinea. *BMC International Health and Human Rights, 12,* 1–18. doi:10.1186/1472-698X-12-10

Kharsany, A. B. M., & Karim, Q. A. (2016). HIV infection and AIDS in sub-Saharan Africa: Current status, challenges, and opportunities. *The Open AIDS Journal, 10,* 34–48. doi:10.2174/1874613601610010034

Mallinson, R. K., & Sibandze, B. T. (2017). Improvisation, partnerships: Learning from our global colleagues. *The Voice of Nursing Leadership, 15*(1), 16–17.

McNeish, H. (2016). Swaziland and HIV: Redrawing what it means to be a man. Retrieved from https://www.aljazeera.com/indepth/features/2016/07/swaziland-hiv-redrawing-means-man-160731091526180.html

Milford, C., Rambally, L., Mantell, J. E., Kelvin, E. A., Mosery, N. F., & Smit, J. A. (2016). Healthcare providers' knowledge, attitudes and practices towards medical male circumcision and their understandings of its partial efficacy in HIV prevention: Qualitative research in KwaZulu-Natal, South Africa. *International Journal of Nursing Studies, 53*, 182–189. doi:10.1016/j.ijnurstu.2015.07.011

Moyo, S., Mhloyi, M., Chevo, T., & Rusinga, O. (2015). Men's attitudes: A hindrance to the demand for voluntary medical male circumcision—A qualitative study in rural Mhondoro-Ngezi, Zimbabwe. *Global Public Health, 10*(5), 708–720. doi:10.1080/17441692.2015.1006241

Smith, A. D. (2012). Why a U.S. circumcision push failed in Swaziland. *PBS Newshour*. Retrieved from http://www.pbs.org/newshour/updates/health-july-dec12-swaziaids_07-05

Upvall, M. J. (2012). Nurse and visiting organization factors for global partnership. In M. J. Upvall & J. M. Lefers (Eds.), *Global health nursing: Building and sustaining partnerships* (pp. 51–59). New York, NY: Springer.

Weaver, J. (1998). Nursing, health, and health care in the international community. In D. J. Mason & J. K. Leavitt (Eds.). *Policy and politics in nursing and health care* (3rd ed.). Philadelphia, PA: W. B. Saunders.

World Health Organization. (2013). World health statistics. Retrieved from http://www.who.int/gho/publications/world-health-st

World Health Organization. (2016). Swaziland. Retrieved from http://www.who.int/countries/swz/en

Providing Access to Clean Water in Rural Nicaragua: A Qualitative Case Study

Johnathan D. Steppe
Mari-Amanda Dyal

Clean, potable drinking water is a fundamental necessity of life. In 2010, the United Nations (UN) identified water and sanitation as an intrinsic human right that is essential to societal development as well as individual and collective health (United Nations [UN], 2010). The Pan American Health Organization (PAHO) has further noted that "no public health intervention has a greater impact on national development and individual and collective health than the provision of drinking water and sanitary excreta disposal" (PAHO, 2011, p. 5). Yet in spite of this recognition, a significant percentage of the world's population still lacks a consistent source of clean water. This disparity is greatest in low- and middle-income countries, with rural communities being at greater risk for water contamination.

The purpose of this chapter is to examine a community health program that is designed to provide sustainable access to clean water in rural Nicaraguan communities. First, the background and significance of clean water access is presented. Next, an overview of clean water initiatives in Nicaragua is provided. Finally, a grassroots clean water program implemented by a nongovernmental organization (NGO) is presented, using a qualitative case study approach. This exemplar case illustrates how one organization was able to design and implement a local solution for a local problem. With respect to global health policy, this chapter highlights how global health initiatives are created and sustained through connections between public policy and community-based interventions.

BACKGROUND AND SIGNIFICANCE

Lack of clean drinking water has serious health implications for individuals and communities worldwide. Water may be contaminated by parasites, bacteria such as *Escherichia coli*, or viruses such as norovirus or rotavirus (Centers for Disease Control and Prevention [CDC], 2015). In addition, persons drinking from unsafe water sources may be exposed to chemical contaminants that may contribute to the development of end-stage renal disease (Wasana et al., 2016; Wimalawansa, 2014, 2016). Undeveloped water sources and improperly stored water also provide potential breeding grounds for mosquitos that can transmit vector-borne diseases such as Zika and dengue (Padmanabha, Soto, Mosquera, Lord, & Lounibos, 2010).

Globally, diarrheal diseases remain the second leading cause of mortality in children under 5 years old (World Health Organization [WHO], 2017). According to WHO, there are approximately 1.7 billion cases of diarrheal disease each year. From these cases, nearly 525,000 children will die from what is most often a preventable and treatable illness (WHO, 2017). The most common cause of diarrheal deaths is ingesting contaminated drinking water, followed by inadequate sanitation and inadequate hand hygiene (Prüss-Ustün et al., 2014). Diarrheal diseases can lead to profound dehydration and can cause or exacerbate malnutrition. Chronic malnutrition has been linked to stunted growth in children, and worldwide, 26% of children under five are considered stunted due to overt or subclinical enteric dysfunction (Mbuya & Humphrey, 2016). In low- and middle-income countries such as Nicaragua, contaminated water sources are one of the major causes of diarrheal disease and enteric disorders, and providing access to safe drinking water is a prevention strategy that has the potential to reduce mortality rates in children under five.

IMPROVING ACCESS TO CLEAN WATER

Given the UN declaration that identified clean water access as a basic human right, it is not surprising that a number of public initiatives have been implemented to increase access. Established in 2000, the

UN's Millennium Development Goals (MDGs) included Goal 7, which outlined specific targets aimed at ensuring environmental sustainability (UN, 2013). Target 7C specifically sought to halve the percentage of the world's population who lacked access to safe drinking water and basic sanitation (UN, 2013). Through a number of sustained initiatives, both public and private, MDG 7C was the first MDG to be met, with 2.1 billion people gaining access to clean water between 1990 and 2010. Organizations that contributed to the attainment of Target 7C included international groups such as PAHO and WHO, larger humanitarian organizations such as United States Agency for International Development (USAID), as well as national, regional, and municipal entities (PAHO, 2011). In addition, smaller humanitarian groups such as NGOs were identified as making significant contributions to increasing global access to clean water. Nevertheless, in spite of such widespread initiatives, approximately 663 million people worldwide still lack access to safe drinking water (UN, 2016). Furthermore, 2.6 billion people are without basic sanitation facilities, a fact which can contribute to or exacerbate contamination of clean water sources (WHO, 2015). Considering these statistics, it is not surprising that the UN included access to clean water and sanitation for all as one of the 2015 Sustainable Development Goals that continue and expand the priorities set forth in the MDGs.

A significant body of evidence demonstrates that interventions that provide better access to clean water and basic sanitation can greatly improve health outcomes related to diarrheal illness. Fewtrell et al. (2005) conducted a systematic review and meta-analysis of research that examined the impact of water, sanitization, and hygiene interventions on the incidence and outcomes of diarrheal illness. Specific to clean water, Fewtrell et al. reviewed interventions that improved water supply and water quality. Water supply interventions were those that provided a new source of water, such as the provision of a new piped water supply or a new household connection to an existing supply. Water quality interventions examined were mainly point-of-use water treatment systems, such as the use of chemical decontaminants, household water filters, boiling water, and solar disinfection (Fewtrell et al., 2005). In addition, several interventions provided improvements to both water supply and water quality. Providing a consistent source of fresh water was found to reduce the need for water storage, a practice that increases the risk of water contamination due to improper storage practices. In addition, systems that disinfected water immediately before drinking (point-of-use decontamination) appeared to be particularly effective at mitigating the risk of diarrheal diseases. According to PAHO (2011), initiatives aimed at improving household water quality appear to have the strongest impact on mitigating mortality and morbidity of diarrheal diseases. Specifically, point-of-use water treatment systems have led to a 35% reduction of diarrheal disease in some areas (Clasen, Nadakatti, & Menon, 2006; Fabiszewski de Aceituno, Stauber, Walters, Meza Sanchez, & Sobsey, 2012; Fewtrell et al., 2005). Furthermore, point-of-use water filtration may be more effective at addressing health outcomes related to clean water access than initiatives that simply increase access to improved water supplies such as indoor plumbing (PAHO, 2011).

A number of studies have demonstrated that point-of-use water filtration systems are effective at improving water quality and reducing the bacteria load of drinking water. Fiore, Minnings, and Fiore (2010) investigated the effectiveness of biosand filters in reducing *E. coli* contamination in the drinking water of rural Nicaraguan households. The study found that the filtration system reduced bacterial load by 80% and that 74% of households using the filter had a significant reduction in *E. coli* colony-forming units. A similar study by Larson, Hansen, Ritz, and Carreño (2017) found that point-of-use water filtration systems significantly reduced the incidence of diarrheal disease in rural Guatemala. Still other studies demonstrated the effectiveness of point-of-care systems at removing pathogens and chemical contaminants in such diverse settings as China, India, South Africa, and Nigeria (Abebe et al., 2014; Barzilay et al., 2011; Cha et al., 2015; Khadse, Kalita, & Labhsetwar, 2012; Smith et al., 2017).

While point-of-use filtration systems appear to be an effective way of improving health through the provision of safe, potable water, there also appear to be limitations to these systems. The various point-of-use technologies require differing degrees of upkeep, which may be challenging for some households to maintain. Pérez-Vidal, Diaz-Gómez, Castellanos-Rozo, and Usaquen-Perilla (2016) noted that the success of point-of-use filters is highly dependent on cleaning and maintenance, and that sustainability of such initiatives depended on training and education of filter recipients. Larson et al. (2017) noted that broken filters contributed to increased incidence of diarrhea, and that some homes lacked flat surfaces on which to place the water filter. Singer, Skinner, and Cantwell (2017) studied the impact of maintenance techniques on the performance of bio-sand water filters, finding that decontamination ability and flow rates were highly dependent on proper maintenance. Finally, Mellor, Abebe, Ehdaie, Dillingham, and Smith (2014) found that improper maintenance of ceramic filters contributed to a decline in the antimicrobial properties of the filter to the point that, after 3 years, the filter became entirely ineffective.

The preceding studies highlight the importance of deliberate and careful planning, implementation, and evaluation of point-of-use water filtration programs. Such programs must not only take into account the immediate benefit of the filters, but the process by which these benefits must be sustained. What follows is a description of a sustainable point-of-use water filtration program that has been implemented by a small NGO working in the rural areas of Nicaragua.

METHODOLOGY

Qualitative case study methodology (QCSM) is a research approach that is well suited to holistic, deep description of a phenomenon that cannot be readily separated from the context in which it occurs. A QCSM approach was chosen because the water filtration program of interest is intimately connected to the communities and culture in which it has been implemented. Furthermore, QCSM allows for complex exploration of the program, which will arguably provide a better understanding of how the program was implemented and sustained.

DELINEATING THE CASE

Both Yin (2009) and Stake (1995), two of the leading theorists of QCSM, agree that defining the case or unit of interest is one of the first steps of the QCSM approach. This study adopted Stake's approach by defining the intrinsic case as a single water safety initiative that has been implemented by an NGO working in the rural communities of Nicaragua. Intrinsic cases are conducted to provide better insight into a particular phenomenon of interest. Intrinsic case studies are not illustrative of a larger theme, but instead provide deep understanding of a specific phenomenon.

DATA COLLECTION

Multiple data collection methods are a hallmark of QCSM. Multiple data sources allow for triangulation of results, which in turn increases the trustworthiness of findings. In this study, data were collected via a semi-structured interview, document review, and field observation of the water filtration program.

The interview was conducted with one of the founders of the water filtration program. During the interview, an initial set of questions were proposed. In addition, follow-up questions were asked to clarify understanding of responses to the initial set of questions. The participant also agreed to provide additional responses during the data analysis phase, so that emerging themes could accurately be identified.

Documents reviewed included information from the program's website, as well as handouts provided during a health summit that was held in one of the communities that had benefited from the water filtration program. In addition, relevant documents and studies were reviewed to provide insight into past and present clean water initiatives that have been implemented in Nicaragua. These documents included public health initiatives implemented by Nicaragua's Ministry of Health (MINSA), as well as information from a number of different private clean water initiatives currently being implemented in rural Nicaragua.

Field observations were conducted in a single rural community in which the water filtration program has been implemented. Home visits were made to nine households that had received filters. During these visits, the filter recipients discussed the benefits of the filter. One recipient demonstrated proper cleaning of the filter. Finally, a demonstration of the filter and presentation on the filter program were given by representatives from the NGO.

CLEAN WATER ACCESS IN RURAL NICARAGUA—A CASE STUDY

As the second poorest country in the western hemisphere, Nicaragua has struggled to provide its people with the basic resources necessary to ensure health and optimal well-being. Political upheavals, war, and natural disasters have made this struggle all the more challenging, although Nicaragua has made great strides in the provision of healthcare through national health programs such as child vaccination initiatives and health education campaigns (Halperin & Garfield, 1982). As previously noted, access to clean water is essential to health, yet historically, many of the rural communities of Nicaragua have lacked a consistent, reliable source of clean water (Halperin & Garfield, 1982). To address this disparity, the Nicaraguan government established Ley 722 in 2010, which enabled the creation of approximately 5,400 community-level water committees that coordinate clean water initiatives with committee stakeholders and external humanitarian groups (Herrera, 2015; PAHO, 2012).

A considerable number of NGOs have sought to improve clean water access for the people of Nicaragua. Indeed, a basic Internet search using the search engine Google and the keywords "clean water Nicaragua" brings up a number of such programs, including Agua para la Vida, Agua Clara, Water for People, WaterAid, and Waves for Water. These programs all have similar missions: To improve access to clean water for the people of Nicaragua through strategies such as distribution of point-of-use water filtration systems. Point-of-use technologies are a common strategy used by NGOs to provide access to clean water for the families and communities of rural Nicaragua. As previously noted, these filters have been shown to improve the safety of drinking water, although their effectiveness depends on the appropriateness of the technology as well as the quality of education and training received by potential users (Pérez-Vidal et al., 2016).

Through these public and private initiatives, Nicaragua has made significant progress toward improving clean water access. Nicaragua succeeded in reaching MDG 7A by reducing, by half, the population of Nicaragua living without clean water access. Yet in spite of this success, significant disparities in the country's rural communities remain. Furthermore, these disparities are more prevalent in poorer homes, where people are more likely to obtain water from unsafe sources (Hong et al., 2013). Weiss, Aw, Urquhart, Galeano, and Rose (2016) used compartment bag testing (CBT) to measure *E. coli* levels in well water in the rural community of Pueblo Nuevo, Nicaragua. The study concluded that water in the community was unsafe and that animal feces was a major source of well contamination. Jordanova et al. (2015) examined access to water, sanitation, and hygiene in Nicaraguan schools. The results of this study found that only 43% of schools had an adequate clean water infrastructure. In low density rural areas, the number of schools with such an infrastructure dropped to 28%.

Clearly, in spite of past progress, further interventions are needed to ensure the people of rural Nicaragua have consistent access to safe drinking water. The following case study explores a clean water program that is currently being implemented in rural communities of Nicaragua. The names of the program, people, and places have been changed to protect anonymity.

WATER FOR NICARAGUA—A POINT-OF-USE WATER FILTRATION PROGRAM

Mike is the cofounder of an NGO that began a water filter program called Water for Nicaragua (WN). Mike's work in Nicaragua began as a journey of self-discovery. After graduating with a history degree in 1998, he embarked on a road trip through Mexico and Central America with two friends. During this time, Mike found himself in Nicaragua, a country that immediately resonated with him. Mike felt a connection to the people of Nicaragua and decided to stay in the country for several months, leaving just weeks before Nicaragua was devastated by Hurricane Mitch. Upon returning to the United States, Mike began teaching English as a second language as a way to stay connected to the Latino community, with whom he felt a strong connection. This connection led Mike back to Nicaragua in 1999, at which time he met the woman who would later become his wife. Mike spent the next several summers in Nicaragua, saving money during the year to fund his trips. In 2002, Mike graduated with a master's degree in social work and began working for the United Way, where he was exposed to a number of social work programs. Mike realized that many of these programs could benefit the people of Nicaragua. Thus, in 2005, Mike left the United Way and returned to Nicaragua, where he hoped to implement his own social program centered on microenterprise development and affordable home ownership. During this time, Mike worked in a number of capacities, including as the editor of a local newspaper and as the head of the social responsibility branch of a major Nicaraguan corporation.

While working in Nicaragua, Mike met Jacob, also from the United States, who was researching the impact of tourism on the communities of Nicaragua. According to Mike, Jacob "opened my eyes to the opportunities within tourism to be a motor for social impact." Together, Mike and Jacob founded an NGO that developed a social enterprise model that combined a sustainable tourism model with community development initiatives. From that model grew a number of social and community development initiatives, including the WN project.

THE CASE FOR CLEAN WATER

Mike's interest in implementing a clean water project came from his observations at health clinics in rural Nicaragua. During his time working in corporate social responsibility outreach, Mike had the opportunity to visit numerous rural health clinics. In Mike's own words:

> As I got to know the rural clinics and their area of influence—there was probably five different clinics there—I realized they were saturated with people every day. There was a nurse and maybe a doctor trying to see 40 up to 50 patients a day. And, as I spent time and got to know what the issues were ... diarrhea, upper respiratory, and other preventable illnesses were clogging up the intake process and care process such that the doctors, nurses, or the staff really couldn't get out in front of it, of those issues.

During this time, a volunteer in Mike's organization had raised funding that he wished to use in a meaningful way. Mike realized that this money could be used to fund a clean water project that had the potential to reduce the prevalence of diarrheal illness in rural communities. In doing so, the project could also ease the burden on rural clinics, which were struggling to care for an overwhelming number of patients. Mike recognized that choosing appropriate technology would be critical to the program's success, so he and his colleagues began research into water filtration systems. This research led them to adopt the Filtron as the system of choice for the WN program.

THE WATER FILTRATION SYSTEM

The Filtron is a point-of-use water filter designed for households in communities with inadequate access to clean water. The technology behind the Filtron is surprisingly simple. Water passes through a specially designed filter that is nested in a plastic collection barrel. The filters are formed from a mixture of clay and sawdust, which is molded into a medium-sized pot. After several days of drying, the filters are fired in a kiln, where the sawdust particles are burned off. The firing process leaves behind a network of tiny pores. These pores are large enough to allow water to pass through, but prevent the passage of parasites. Furthermore, each filter is treated with a colloidal silver solution, giving the filter antimicrobial properties. The collection barrel allows for easy storage of filtered water, which is protected from recontamination by a plastic cover. The water is then dispensed via a spigot installed at the bottom of the collection barrel.

The Filtron water filters are produced by a company in Nicaragua that was started by the NGO, Potters for Peace. Using a local company aligned with Mike's belief that local problems necessitated local solutions. By using a Nicaraguan-based company, Mike felt that the project further supported the people of Nicaragua and the ultimate sustainability of the water project. Mike noted that other filter technologies were considered. These included biosand filters and Sawyer-type filters. However, Mike's organization found that many of these filters were not appropriate for their target population. For example, biosand filters require users to establish and maintain a layer of bacteria as part of the filter upkeep. Mike felt that this level of maintenance was inappropriate given the average education level in rural Nicaraguan communities. In addition, the biosand technologies that Mike observed in Nicaragua required the use of a significant amount of concrete. This concrete increases the weight of the filter, which in turn makes delivery of the filter to remote communities a greater challenge. Ultimately, Mike felt that the Filtron system offered a simple technology that could be readily implemented and maintained by community residents. In addition, the lighter weight of the Filtron system made it easier for the WN staff to deliver the filters to even the remotest rural communities.

IMPLEMENTING AND EVALUATING THE WATER FILTER PROGRAM

Before implementing the WN program, Mike sought input from experts at the Center for Global Safe Water, Sanitation, and Hygiene (CGSW), which is attached to the Rollins School of Health at Emory University. CGSW has experience working with larger NGOs such as United Nations Children's Fund (UNICEF) and Cooperative for Assistance and Relief Everywhere (CARE). Mike was advised that the success of a water filter program depended on the level of commitment of the local partners and the extent to which the program fostered ownership, provided education, and established effective evaluation and follow-up procedures. From this advice, Mike's organization recognized the need to build in each of these components into the WN program.

ESTABLISHING OWNERSHIP

According to Mike, WN begins implementation of the water filter program by building relationships with a community and its leaders. WN then evaluates interest in the water filtration program, recognizing that ownership can be enhanced by implementing projects that are grounded in the priorities of the community. Mike's organization recognized that the majority of potential WN beneficiaries would not have the financial means to purchase a water filter, and so ownership would need to be established through a different mechanism. Recognizing that simply giving filters away would not foster ownership, Mike and his colleagues designed a program by which community members could earn a water filter by completing 16 hours of community service work. The nature of the community service work centered on supporting or establishing community assets such as parks, roads, schools, and clinics, resources that could benefit everyone in the community. This community-asset approach also aligned with the NGO's broader goals of facilitating community development. In Mike's own words:

> We can use ... we can catalyze community service in support of community assets. And we felt that two day's work would be the equivalent of what the cost of the filter would be.... And a lot of the community projects we coordinate with them—because a lot of times they are like "oh, what can we do?" And so, the work of a social worker is to kind of nudge or glean out these ideas, and not tell people what they should be doing, but just ask them the questions. "What's important to you? What do you see as priorities?" So you do a consensus building exercise, and that's how community projects were identified. And they were typically projects that families couldn't do alone. And so we got people together improving the roads, the drainage on the roads, community cleanups, improvements at the school, things of that nature.

Mike's organization has found that this investment of time facilitates recipient ownership of the filter, and that very rarely have they seen the filters discarded, sold, given away, or used in an inappropriate manner, such as for storage or for a planter.

During field observations, one author noted that all of the filters were being used for their intended purpose, that of water filtration. Usually, the filters were placed in a prominent location—for example, on a table at the center of the living area or kitchen—and several of the observed filters had been decorated with hand-knitted covers or ribbons. Mike stated that such decorations were not only common but the additional covering provided another layer of protection from contamination. The filters appeared in good condition, and some of them had been in use for several years. When asked about the filter, one resident commented that she was proud of her filter because it represented the family's hard work and dedication. Her words suggested that the required community service hours contributed to a sense of pride and ownership in the water filter.

EDUCATION

In addition to the 16 required community service hours, recipients of a WN water filter must attend a mandatory training session over the proper use and maintenance of the Filtron. This training session is conducted on the day the filters arrive and lasts approximately 45 minutes. Furthermore, water filter recipients must also attend a health and hygiene seminar that covers topics such as handwashing and maintaining a healthy and clean home environment. Mike noted that this seminar allows his organization to go beyond clean water to address related health topics that further contribute to the foundational concepts of water, sanitation, and hygiene. In addition, because the seminars are scheduled in the nearest health clinic, water filter recipients who may not have been aware of clinic services are exposed and subsequently connected to this important community asset. According to Mike, the seminars can thus be a bridge between community members, not only by enhancing education but by fostering community connections between residents, and between residents and community resources.

While conducting field observations, one of the authors visited homes of nine different water filter recipients. On two of these visits, the homeowners demonstrated how they cleaned the filter each week, using a small plastic brush that they stored close to the filter. The cleaning process was simple and only required access to a brush, some clean water, and occasionally some type of disinfectant such as chlorine. The fact that recipients were able to "teach back" the cleaning process supported the effectiveness of WN's education process.

EVALUATION AND FOLLOW-UP

Of the components of the WN program, Mike acknowledged that evaluation and follow-up has been the most challenging piece and is a phase of the program that is still being refined. When first implementing the program in a new community, the organization first collects baseline demographic data from residents who express interest in receiving a water filter. According to Mike, there is a dearth of community-level data in Nicaragua, so Mike's organization recognized an opportunity to collect some of that local data that could be used to evaluate the program's effectiveness. Once baseline data have been collected and filters have been distributed, the WN staff schedule follow-up visits to the homes of filter recipients. A total of three follow-up visits are scheduled during the first year of ownership. These visits occur 1, 3, and 6 months after receipt of the filter. In addition, WN schedules at least one home visit during the second year of filter ownership. Mike noted that WN commits to at least 2 years of engagement with the community to adequately monitor program effectiveness. During the follow-up visits, WN staff evaluate how the filter is being used, how the filter has impacted the health and well-being of filter recipients, and how well the recipients understand the function and proper maintenance of the filter. Recipients are asked about episodes of diarrhea and other illnesses, as well as about their family's general sense of well-being. WN staff also evaluate the family's living conditions, noting if there have been any noticeable improvements to cleanliness in the home. Mike's organization also recognizes the need of long-term program evaluation. According to Mike:

> We are now getting to the point that people have had the filters long enough that the filters are reaching the end of their life cycle, because they don't work forever. Some water has more turbidity than others, some filters are trying to serve a family of ten, while other filters only serve a family of two or three. So, it's hard to generalize how long a filter will last ... and I always felt that one of the best reflections of sustainability of this program, or success in that regard, would be a family's willingness to pay for a replacement. Because financial resources are so scarce.

WN is currently working with local partners, such as community banks, to create a process by which community residents could finance and obtain replacement filters. Mike noted that a willingness to do so would reflect the level of value and ownership that residents have for the program. Still, Mike acknowledged that there can be circumstances in which families are unable to earn filters through money or community service. For example, older families with chronic illnesses may lack the ability to earn money and may also be physically unable to participate in community service. Mike shared that the WN staff are currently investigating alternative processes through which such families could still receive a filter.

DISCUSSION

To date, WN has implemented their water filtration program in approximately 15 communities and in nearly 2,000 households. Mike estimated that the WN program has benefited 7,000 residents in communities ranging from the Pacific coast of Nicaragua, to the country's northern mountains, and even to the eastern autonomous regions that border the Caribbean. During data analysis, three key themes emerged that appear to drive the philosophy and success of the WN program. These themes were: (a) community connections, (b) community development, and (c) sustainability.

COMMUNITY CONNECTIONS

When Mike first started working in Nicaragua, he founded a newspaper that he named *La Puente*, or *The Bridge*. This name reflects the WN approach with communities, in that one of its major goals is to bridge connections between community residents and each other, and between residents and their community resources. Mike's work with the United Way and his connections with other global aid organizations has informed his viewpoint, and he seems to deeply value social connections, connections through which the work of the WN program is accomplished and sustained. As noted above, the first step of the WN program is to build relationships with local communities. As the program is implemented, the community service component brings community members together, working for the good of the community as a whole. This connection can be particularly beneficial for isolated residents, who may become more engaged with their community through such work. Mike finds that once these residents are engaged, they often remain engaged and become active in their community. Mike noted that the clean water filtration program is a catalyst for broader changes, changes that enhance the social fabric of communities.

COMMUNITY DEVELOPMENT

As Mike noted, what began as a simple water filtration project ultimately transformed into the foundation of a broader community development program. The mechanism by which recipients earned the water filters directly contributed to the development of community-based assets, which benefited the community as a whole. In addition, Mike's organization offers opportunities for individuals and families to earn other health-related improvements for their homes. For example, residents may complete additional community service hours to receive an improved stove or outdoor oven. Community service hours can also be used to earn installation of a concrete floor in a family's home or the rooms of the home can be treated with a sticky paint that attracts, catches, and kills mosquitos. However, to receive any of these projects, the home must first earn and maintain a water filter for the home. Interestingly, this structure mirrors the UN position that the provision of clean water and basic sanitation is essential for all other aspects of community development. Given Mike's previous experience with USAID and his knowledge and connections with other global health players, it is not surprising that the WN structure reflects broader global health policies. It appears that the WN program has benefited from an informed knowledge of both global health policy and best practice guidelines.

SUSTAINABILITY

A shift toward designing and implementing global policies that emphasize sustainability is evident with the establishment of the UN's Sustainable Development Goals, which grew out of the previously enacted MDGs. The choice to reference sustainability in naming the goals is clearly intentional and reflects a global orientation toward ensuring that policy supports sustainable change.

The WN program integrates principles of sustainability at each level of the program. Initially, the organization assesses the needs and priorities of the community, thereby ensuring that the program will be grounded in the community's priorities. By establishing ownership, residents are more likely to maintain their water filters, and thus can enjoy long-term benefits of clean water access. Appropriate and sustained education also increases the chances for long-term success; as previously noted, proper maintenance of filtration technology is a critical component to the success of clean water initiatives. Finally, Mike's organization enhances sustainability through a lasting commitment to the communities with whom they work. Mike argued that simply distributing filters is not enough to achieve lasting improvements to health. Instead, groups should partner with communities to build knowledge, value, and commitment to the significant health benefits associated with clean water.

CONCLUSION

It is clear that the clean water program examined in the preceding pages was informed by global health policies and grounded in best practices established by key public health organizations. Continued progress toward meeting water safety goals is dependent on organizations, both public and private, that can create innovative interventions that are not only effective but also sustainable. Humanitarian efforts by large and small entities can benefit from sound global policies, which can provide a guiding framework for groups wishing to achieve meaningful, long-lasting global change.

REFERENCES

Abebe, L. S., Smith, J. A., Narkiewicz, S., Oyanedel-Craver, V., Conaway, M., Singo, A., ... Dillingham, R. (2014). Ceramic water filters impregnated with silver nanoparticles as a point-of-use water-treatment intervention for HIV-positive individuals in Limpopo Province, South Africa: A pilot study of technological performance and human health benefits. *Journal of Water and Health, 12*(2), 288–300. doi:10.2166/wh.2013.185

Barzilay, E. J., Aghoghovbia, T. S., Blanton, E. M., Akinpelumi, A. A., Coldiron, M. E., Akinfolayan, O., ... Quick, R. (2011). Diarrhea prevention in people living with HIV: An evaluation of a point-of-use water quality intervention in Lagos, Nigeria. *AIDS Care, 23*(3), 330–339. doi:10.1080/09540121.2010.507749

Centers for Disease Control and Prevention. (2015). *Diseases and contaminants.* Atlanta, GA: Author. Retrieved from https://www.cdc.gov/healthywater/drinking/private/wells/disease/norovirus.html

Cha, S., Kang, D., Tuffuor, B., Lee, G., Cho, J., Chung, J., ... Oh, C. (2015). The effect of improved water supply on diarrhea prevalence of children under five in the Volta region of Ghana: A cluster-randomized controlled trial. *International Journal of Environmental Research and Public Health, 12*(10), 12127–12143. doi:10.3390/ijerph121012127

Clasen, T., Nadakatti, S., & Menon, S. (2006). Microbiological performance of a water treatment unit designed for household use in developing countries. *Tropical Medicine & International Health, 11*(9), 1399–1405. doi:10.1111/j.1365-3156.2006.01699.x

Fabiszewski de Aceituno, A. M., Stauber, C. E., Walters, A. R., Meza Sanchez, R. E., & Sobsey, M. D. (2012). A randomized controlled trial of the plastic-housing

BioSand filter and its impact on diarrheal disease in Copan, Honduras. *The American Journal of Tropical Medicine and Hygiene, 86*(6), 913–921. doi:10.4269/ajtmh.2012.11-0066

Fewtrell, L., Kaufmann, R. B., Kay, D., Enanoria, W., Haller, L., & Colford, J. M. (2005). Water, sanitation, and hygiene interventions to reduce diarrhoea in less developed countries: A systematic review and meta-analysis. *The Lancet Infectious Diseases. 5*(1), 42–52. doi:10.1016/S1473-3099(04)01253-8

Fiore, M., Minnings, K., & Fiore, L. (2010). Assessment of biosand filter performance in rural communities in southern coastal Nicaragua: An evaluation of 199 households. *Rural & Remote Health, 10*(3), 1483.

Halperin, D. C., & Garfield, R. (1982). Developments in health care in Nicaragua. *The New England Journal of Medicine, 307*(6), 388–392. doi:10.1056/NEJM198208053070634

Herrera, R. S. (2015). *Nicaragua: How much longer will the country's water last?* Retrieved from www.envio.org.ni/articulo/4895

Hong, Y., Bain, R., Bartram, J., Gundry, S., Pedley, S., & Wright, J. (2013). Water safety and inequality in access to drinking-water between rich and poor households. *Environmental Science & Technology, 47*(3), 1222–1230. doi:10.1021/es303345p

Jordanova, T., Cronk, R., Obando, W., Medina, O. Z., Kinoshita, R., & Bartram, J. (2015). Water, sanitation, and hygiene in schools in low socio-economic regions in Nicaragua: A cross-sectional survey. *International Journal of Environmental Research and Public Health, 12*(6), 6197–6217. doi:10.3390/ijerph120606197

Khadse, G. K., Kalita, M. D., & Labhsetwar, P. K. (2012). Change in drinking water quality from source to point-of-use and storage: A case study from Guwahati, India. *Environmental Monitoring and Assessment, 184*(9), 5343–5361. doi:10.1007/s10661-011-2344-8

Larson, K. L., Hansen, C., Ritz, M., & Carreño, D. (2017). Acceptance and impact of point-of-use water filtration systems in rural Guatemala. *Journal of Nursing Scholarship, 49*(1), 96–102. doi:10.1111/jnu.12260

Mbuya, M. N., & Humphrey, J. H. (2016). Preventing environmental enteric dysfunction through improved water, sanitation and hygiene: An opportunity for stunting reduction in developing countries. *Maternal & Child Nutrition, 12*(S1), 106–120. doi:10.1111/mcn.12220

Mellor, J., Abebe, L., Ehdaie, B., Dillingham, R., & Smith, J. (2014). Modeling the sustainability of a ceramic water filter intervention. *Water Research, 49*, 286–299. doi:10.1016/j.watres.2013.11.035

Padmanabha, H., Soto, E., Mosquera, M., Lord, C. C., & Lounibos, L. P. (2010). Ecological links between water storage behaviors and *Aedes aegypti* production: Implications for dengue vector control in variable climates. *EcoHealth, 7*(1), 78–90. doi:10.1007/s10393-010-0301-6

Pan American Health Organization. (2011). *Water and sanitation: Evidence for public policies focused on human rights and public health results*. Retrieved from http://www.paho.org/hq/index.php?option=com_docman&task=doc _download&gid=17606&Itemid=270&lang=en.

Pan American Health Organization. (2012). *Nicaragua*. Washington, DC: Author. Retrieved from http://www.paho.org/salud-en-las-americas-2012/index .php?option=com_docman&task=doc_view&gid=140&Itemid

Pérez-Vidal, A., Diaz-Gómez, J., Castellanos-Rozo, J., & Usaquen-Perilla, O. L. (2016). Long-term evaluation of the performance of four point-of-use water filters. *Water Research, 98,* 176–182. doi:10.1016/j.watres.2016.04.016

Prüss-Ustün, A., Bartram, J., Clasen, T., Colford, J. M., Cumming, O., Curtis, V., ... Cairncross, S. (2014). Burden of disease from inadequate water, sanitation and hygiene in low- and middle-income settings: A retrospective analysis of data from 145 countries. *Tropical Medicine & International Health, 19*(8), 894–905. doi:10.1111/tmi.12329

Singer, S., Skinner, B., & Cantwell, R. E. (2017). Impact of surface maintenance on BioSand filter performance and flow. *Journal of Water & Health, 15*(2), 262–272. doi:10.2166/wh.2017.129

Smith, K., Li, Z., Chen, B., Liang, H., Zhang, X., Xu, R., ... Liu, S. (2017). Comparison of sand-based water filters for point-of-use arsenic removal in China. *Chemosphere, 168,* 155–162. doi:10.1016/j.chemosphere.2016.10.021

Stake, R. E. (1995). *The art of case study research*. Thousand Oaks, CA: Sage.

United Nations. (2010). *The human right to water and sanitation*. Retrieved from http://www.un.org/es/comun/docs/?symbol=A/RES/64/292&lang=E

United Nations. (2013). *MDG 7: Ensure environmental sustainability*. Retrieved from http://www.who.int/topics/millennium_development_goals/mdg7/en/

United Nations. (2016). *Water*. Retrieved from http://www.un.org/en/sections/ issues-depth/water/

Wasana, H., Aluthpatabendi, D., Kularatne, W., Wijekoon, P., Weerasooriya, R., & Bandara, J. (2016). Drinking water quality and chronic kidney disease of unknown etiology (CKDu): Synergic effects of fluoride, cadmium and hardness of water. *Environmental Geochemistry and Health, 38*(1), 157–168. doi:10.1007/s10653-015-9699-7

Weiss, P., Aw, T. G., Urquhart, G. R., Galeano, M. R., & Rose, J. B. (2016). Well water quality in rural Nicaragua using a low-cost bacterial test and microbial source tracking. *Journal of Water and Health, 14*(2), 199–207. doi:10.2166/wh.2015.075

Wimalawansa, S. (2014). Escalating chronic kidney diseases of multi-factorial origin in Sri Lanka: Causes, solutions, and recommendations. *Environmental Health and Preventive Medicine, 19*(6), 375-394. doi:10.1007/s12199-014-0395-5

Wimalawansa, S. (2016). The role of ions, heavy metals, fluoride, and agrochemicals: Critical evaluation of potential aetiological factors of chronic kidney disease of multifactorial origin (CKDmfo/CKDu) and recommendations for its eradication. *Environmental Geochemistry and Health, 38*(3), 639-678. doi:10.1007/s10653-015-9768-y

World Health Organization. (2015). *Lack of sanitation for 2.4 billion people is undermining health improvements.* Retrieved from http://www.who.int/mediacentre/news/releases/2015/jmp-report/en/

World Health Organization. (2017). *Diarrhoeal disease.* Retrieved from http://www.who.int/mediacentre/factsheets/fs330/en/

Yin, R. K. (2009). *Case study research: Design and methods* (4th ed.). Thousand Oaks, CA: Sage.

Exemplars of Health Policy
Related to Specific Conditions

Global Health for Transgender Individuals

Amy P. Roach

This chapter focuses on the issues experienced by the global transgender health population. A background is provided on transgender healthcare and current published studies focusing on transgender health outcomes. Additionally, a description is given on policies and legislation that protects transgender individuals in certain countries. The gaps in transgender health and research are also discussed in an effort to bring awareness and visibility to this marginalized and stigmatized population.

GLOBAL HEALTH FOR TRANSGENDER INDIVIDUALS

There are an estimated 25 million individuals who identify as transgender in the world (Reisner et al., 2016). *Transgender* is an umbrella term used to identify individuals outside the gender binary of man and woman. Within this umbrella, terms such as male-to-female (MTF) transgender, female-to-male (FTM) transgender, gender queer, and gender nonbinary may be used by gender minority individuals. The most commonly used gender nonbinary terms are MTF and FTM transgender. These identifiers are used for individuals who experience gender outside of the sex they were assigned at birth (Pega & Veale, 2015). An individual expresses his or her gender through outward appearance and mannerisms (Pega & Veale, 2015). While gender has become more fluid over the last few decades, particularly in the United States, there are still established gender norms and roles that are upheld by many cultures and societies worldwide.

For instance, many countries and cultures maintain gender norms within families and society where a woman has her roles in the home caring for her family and a man has his roles to provide financial support for his family, as well as how they present themselves to others. With these gender roles in place, an individual who experiences gender differently may have a difficult time integrating into society, being accepted, and receiving adequate healthcare. This chapter provides the reader with an understanding of the issues transgender individuals face globally along with how healthcare is accessed and provided to this vulnerable population.

BACKGROUND ON TRANSGENDERISM

Transgender is an umbrella term encompassing a variety of gender expressions that are outside the gender binary or incongruent with an individual's sex assigned at birth. While many in the world identify with their birth sex (known as cisgender individuals), there are others who have a normal variation of their gender expression. In the past, this variation was considered a mental illness, and this illness can still be found in the *Diagnostic and Statistical Manual of Mental Disorders*, 5th ed. (*DSM-5*); however, the current philosophy of treatment by the World Professional Association for Transgender Health (WPATH) includes providing care that is safe and effective while achieving an overall enhanced quality of life (World Professional Association for Transgender Health [WPATH], 2011). Many practitioners provide care to transgender individuals in an effort to integrate the individual into society and improve self-worth and self-esteem (WPATH, 2011). However, there exist inequities and disparities for the transgender population worldwide (Reisner et al., 2016).

Pega and Veale (2015) outline how social determinants of health, as recognized by the World Health Organization (WHO), have affected gender minorities. For instance, transgender individuals face health inequalities related to access and qualified, informed care across the globe (Pega & Veale, 2015). Healthcare providers are uninformed or lack education on how to safely and effectively care for the needs of the transgender population (Grant et al., 2011). In conjunction with social stigma, prejudice, and discrimination, transgender individuals face overwhelming barriers to care that lead to poor health outcomes (Grant et al., 2011). Based on this knowledge, Pega and Veale (2015) identify gender identity as a social determinant of health as this population endures social exclusion, high rates of suicide and mental illness, exposure to violence and discrimination, as well as inherent transphobia in cultural structures. They argue that while gender identity does not "determine health," the social manifestations of gender discrimination and stigma "influence health" (Pega & Veale, 2015, p. e59).

While the abovementioned literature provides a condensed overview of the issues transgender individuals experience, there is historical, social, and political significance to the issues that they have and are faced by this population. The transgender population has been identified as a subset of the lesbian, gay, bisexual, transgender, queer, and intersex (LGBTQI) umbrella. However, the social and health needs of the transgender population are significantly different than the sexual identities within the LGBTQI umbrella. For instance, some transgender individuals desire their outward appearance to match their internal gender expression, which requires medical intervention with hormones and surgery. This is typically not the case for sexual minorities. Additionally, social stigma related to restrooms, housing, and employment are still active in today's modern social settings for transgender individuals, whereas for sexual minorities, while not completely liberated socially and politically, more movement has been seen toward equality with their heterosexual counterparts.

Briefly, medical therapy for transgender individuals may seem complicated and dangerous for healthcare professionals who are unfamiliar with current interventions; however, WPATH (2011) has outlined standards of care for the transgender population which identify the current safe and effective treatments to meet the needs of a transgender individual's gender expression. These interventions include hormone replacement therapy (HRT), surgical intervention, mental health, voice therapy, and preventative care.

HRT may include masculinizing hormones (i.e., testosterone) for FTM transgender people or feminizing hormones (i.e., estrogen) for MTF transgender people, and requires physical and laboratory assessments to ensure the client is healthy to receive the therapy (WPATH, 2011). It is also important for the prescribing provider to understand the risk/benefit ratio of the intervention for safety and efficacy (WPATH, 2011). While some transgender individuals will be satisfied with only HRT, others will desire surgical intervention to modify their body to match their desired gender expression.

Gender-confirming surgeries (GCS) are surgical interventions to help "alleviate [transgender individuals'] gender dysphoria" (WPATH, 2011, p. 54). Gender dysphoria is the distress a person experiences due to the discrepancy between a person's birth sex and gender expression (WPATH, 2011). And it is important to note that all client care should be individualized for the person's needs and desires, as no two transgender individuals will require the same interventions or care. GCS can provide a level of comfort for transgender individuals in their sexual lives and in other aspects of their lives. GCS can include breast or chest surgery, genital surgery, facial reconstruction, and other aesthetic procedures (WPATH, 2011).

Additionally, mental health is a priority area of a person's health that needs to be addressed for the transgender person. Mental healthcare helps a transgender individual reconcile their birth sex with their gender expression, become comfortable with their gender expression, and provide interventional care for mental illnesses such as depression, anxiety, and substance abuse (WPATH, 2011). Mental health providers may also act as a gatekeeper for transgender clients to receive HRT, as many endocrinologists or prescribing providers require mental health assessments prior to initiating HRT. It is important for transgender individuals to have well-informed, qualified, and culturally sensitive mental health professionals to provide care.

Transgender individuals, when attempting to seek healthcare, whether it be for one's gender identity or for illness, injury, or preventative care, receive a brief overview of gender-confirming therapies and a description of the barriers to care. In the United States, there have been two large-scale studies published that have not been replicated elsewhere in the world. Both were initiated by the National Center for Transgender Equality. These studies were completed 5 years apart and resulted in very similar statistics despite different sample sizes and the increase in health insurance coverage for transgender individuals under the Affordable Care Act.

In 2011, Grant et al. surveyed 6,450 transgender individuals, and in 2016, James et al. surveyed 27,715 participants. This many transgender study participants is unprecedented anywhere in the world and has provided rich statistical evidence of the barriers and prejudice transgender individuals face daily. For instance, James et al. (2016) found that violence, prejudice, and mistreatment has continued significantly since the Grant et al. (2011) survey, with 46% having been verbally harassed in the last year and 47% having been sexually assaulted at some point in their life. In regard to healthcare, the statistics seem overwhelming, with poor access to care related to insurance (25%), encounters with uninformed providers (50%), and negative experiences with providers (33%; Grant et al., 2011; James et al., 2016). Furthermore, 40% had attempted suicide in their lifetime, which is nine times higher than the U.S. population (4.6%; Grant et al., 2011; James et al., 2016).

With such alarming statistics, it is conceivable that a priority in healthcare would be to improve access and quality of care for this marginalized population, at least in the U.S. healthcare arena; however, this is far from the case with the current political administration. Yet, there have been pushbacks by transgender advocates to improve insurance coverage and decrease discrimination in public settings for transgender individuals (National Center for Transgender Equality, 2017). Unfortunately, poor healthcare and experiences of discrimination seem to be a reoccurring theme across the world in regard to this population. The following sections provide an in-depth look at the global healthcare arena, including the United States, for transgender individuals.

GLOBAL OVERVIEW OF TRANSGENDER HEALTHCARE

Reisner et al. (2016) identified how transgender health issues are a global health burden, based on the social determinants of health associated with gender identity and the multifactorial health inequities among this vulnerable population. Reisner et al. (2016) cited stigma and discrimination as issues that lead to poor health outcomes for transgender individuals worldwide. Globally, the issues the transgender population face are similar, including prejudice from society and healthcare workers, poor access to informed care, and lack of financial support for healthcare needs (Reisner et al., 2016). Additionally, the lack of transgender research was found to be a major hindrance to understanding the difficulty transgender individuals have as the United States was the only country found in Reisner et al.'s (2016) literature review of globally published research that had more than six studies related to transgender health. With this knowledge, it is essential that the global platform of transgender advocates, providers, and researchers aim to increase visibility and improve health outcomes for transgender individuals.

The outcomes that Reisner et al. (2016) found among the published global transgender health literature included "mental health, sexual and reproductive health, substance abuse, violence and victimization, stigma and discrimination, and general health outcomes" (p. 422). Among the literature, it was identified that transgender health outcomes resulted in high levels of depression, anxiety, and suicide as well as incidence of HIV and sexually transmitted infections (STIs; Reisner et al., 2016). With the prevalence of violence and stigma, transgender individuals have been found to participate in employment that is unsafe (i.e., sex work) and exhibit poor coping mechanisms. For instance, alcohol, drug, and tobacco use has been found to be an issue among the transgender population in relation to minority stress associated with one's gender identity (Reisner et al., 2016). Additionally, employment for transgender individuals has been challenging as 30% of participants in the James et al. (2016) study were fired or experienced mistreatment due to their gender identity. This has led to a high prevalence of transgender individuals partaking in sex work for a means of income, which results in high rates of HIV and STIs as well as physical and sexual assault (James et al., 2016).

Furthermore, mental health issues are predominant across the literature for the transgender population (Reisner et al., 2016). Grant et al. (2011) and James et al. (2016) found high levels of psychological distress related to gender identity among the 35,000 participants in the two U.S. large-scale surveys. Reisner et al. (2016) were able to see the alarming prevalence of mental illness globally across studies, particularly incidences of depression. However, Reisner et al. (2016) identified gaps in the available literature related to posttraumatic stress disorder (PTSD), eating disorders, and perceived body image.

There are many studies that have focused on HIV prevalence, particularly among transgender women of color in the United States. One interesting article written by Terrell (2011) identifies transgender women of color as experiencing a double burden due to their minority gender identity in combination with their racial and ethnic minority status. With these two minority identifications, the incidence of low employment rates, poor healthcare coverage, and high rates of HIV are overwhelming. The stress transgender women of color experience related to their minority status results in a sense of fear that has led to an underreporting of the violence they experience from the public along with the violence and discrimination they experience from police and healthcare providers (Grant et al., 2011; James et al., 2016; Terrell, 2011). Therefore, again, the need for visibility and awareness of transgender issues is apparent, even among the professions who are named to protect and serve (i.e., police and healthcare professions). Additionally, Reisner et al. (2016) identified the need for more research on transgender men related to HIV and STIs, as current research has focused on transgender women.

Lastly, Reisner et al. (2016) recommend the need for several actions to improve health outcomes and bring awareness to the transgender population. One of these recommendations is identifying how marginalized social and economic populations link to certain health indicators (Reisner et al., 2016). Additionally, there is a need for more longitudinal and intervention-based studies as currently many studies focus on cross-sectional time frames and survey type methods (Reisner et al., 2016).

Furthermore, there is a dire need to accurately count the number of transgender individuals globally. While there is an estimation of 0.3% to 0.5% of the global population (roughly 25 million) identify as transgender, the need to assess the health inequities among this population is important to ascertain the knowledge needed to improve health outcomes (Reisner et al., 2016). Additionally, Reisner et al. (2016) recommend developing new frameworks to guide health research for transgender participants. For instance, Reisner et al. (2016) argue that gender and sex are consolidated in research currently as opposed to understanding the difference between sex and gender and the issues that are related to each concept. The current models used in transgender research include minority stress, human rights approach, and gender affirmation. However, the need for analyzing gender, the interchange of gender and sex, and the social determinants of health related to gender were recognized with the recommendation to utilize a model that identifies how sex and gender affect health risks and resiliency (Reisner et al., 2016). This type of framework would investigate how social structures and power lead to health outcomes. Because gender minorities have multifactorial inequities in politics, health, and society, this type of model would be beneficial to understand the layers of issues transgender individuals experience.

Other recommendations Reisner et al. (2016) offer for global transgender health include condemning widespread discrimination, initiating protective laws, and instituting gender rights among international human rights. Research should move to collect evidence for practice, along with the integration of transgender content among formal healthcare training programs, which will improve understanding of transgender needs and issues (Grant et al., 2011; James et al., 2016; Reisner et al., 2016). Lastly, Reisner et al. (2016) recommend utilizing participatory action as a method of research which will enhance sustainability among the transgender population along with creating a sense of inclusion by participating in research as opposed to being the subject of research.

Another issue to consider for transgender healthcare is the diagnosing tools used worldwide. In the United States, the *DSM-5* is utilized to classify mental disorders for all clients; and within this system, gender dysphoria is used to diagnose transgender clients who have experienced distress related to their gender identity (Güldenring, 2015). While the mental health community has taken the stance to use this diagnosis to treat transgender clients in the effort to improve quality of life and integrate the individual into society as the desired gender, the use of gender dysphoria as a diagnosis continues to pathologize nonconforming gender identities (Güldenring, 2015).

In other parts of the world, particularly in Germany, the *International Statistical Classification of Diseases and Related Health Problems (ICD)* is utilized in a similar fashion to the *DSM-5*. The *ICD* is currently in its 10th revision and is published by WHO (Güldenring, 2015). Within *ICD-10*, the current diagnosis for transgender clients is gender identity disorder, which continues a similar path to *DSM-5*, as it pathologizes transgenderism (Güldenring, 2015). Currently, 55.8% of mental health providers worldwide identify the need to unpathologize transgenderism, which will, in turn, help to remove the stigma associated socially, medically, and politically for nonconforming gender identities (Güldenring, 2015). However, there is a hesitancy to remove the diagnostic classification system for transgender clients due to the potential for lack of healthcare insurance coverage without a proper diagnosis. As the eleventh revision of *ICD* is published in 2018, a debate between stakeholders continues regarding gender identity disorder (Güldenring, 2015). Despite the debate, WHO will convert gender identity disorder to gender incongruence in *ICD-11* (Balakrishnan, 2016; Güldenring, 2015). With this transition to a diagnosis of gender incongruence, the treatment goals recommended by WHO will mimic *DSM-5*, which is to provide care that will meet the needs and experiences of the transgender individual while ensuring health equity for the vulnerable population (Güldenring, 2015; Thomas et al., 2017).

TRANSGENDER HEALTHCARE IN SELECT COUNTRIES

With the foundation laid for understanding the barriers and issues to healthcare for transgender individuals, the following sections discuss transgender health and research in several areas around the world. The sections feature Australia, New Zealand, India, Canada, and the United States, including a study on transgender individuals living in rural areas.

AUSTRALIA AND NEW ZEALAND

Riggs, Ansara, and Treharne (2015) performed a literature review of published Australian research on transgender health as well as created a model to utilize when conducting research on this population. Through the literature review, Riggs et al. (2015) found very little Australian-driven research on transgender mental health. However, Riggs et al. (2015) did find that what has been published coincided with findings across the globe from Grant et al. (2011) and James et al. (2016) in that discrimination, access to gender-specific healthcare (i.e., HRT and GCS), and access to a connected community were important in how health was affected for this population. Additionally, depression was a major mental health concern for Australian transgender individuals, and the common causal experience among the population was occurrences of discrimination. Moreover, it was found that an individual's age also affected one's mental health, as the older adults in the studies were found to be mentally healthier than the younger adults (Riggs et al., 2015). Also, the ability to receive gender-confirming interventions (i.e., HRT and GCS) allowed an individual to have improved self-esteem and mental health, along with belonging to a community of accepting and supportive people (Riggs et al., 2015).

Riggs et al. (2015) identified theoretical frameworks after a review of the literature that were important to utilize when addressing research involving transgender participants. The frameworks Riggs et al. (2015) featured were cisgenderism and decompensation. Cisgenderism is conceptualized as pathologizing gender nonconformity and misgendering transgender individuals, whether it is socially or medically, and decompensation is noted to be when a transgender individual becomes vulnerable to the affect cisgenderism plays on the person (Riggs et al., 2015). With these two frameworks combined, Riggs et al. (2015) argue for the use of the Model of Transgender Mental Health in Australia, where the impact of cisgenderism, or discrimination, prejudice, and stigma, lead to an individual's inability to compensate mentally, causing depression and other poor mental health outcomes. Lastly, Riggs et al. (2015) defend the use of the Model of Transgender Mental Health in Australia as a way to improve evidence-based practice for transgender individuals, along with advocating for the removal of a pathological diagnosis of dysphoria related to a person's gender identity.

In New Zealand, there is an effort to account for transgender individuals within the country's census more accurately than current standards. No other country is known to have a statistical standard for gender identity

(Pega, Reisner, Sell, & Veale, 2017). The Institute of Medicine (IOM, 2011) currently is prioritizing data collection related to gender identity for transgender health research. This priority is also emphasized by Reisner et al. (2016) in an effort to improve health outcomes for the transgender population.

New Zealand has made strides in transgender rights by legally protecting gender nonconformity from discrimination and funding four GCS every 2 years (Pega et al., 2017). To accurately count transgender people in New Zealand, the government developed the statistical standard for gender identity for classifcation purposes, which was initiated in 2015 (Pega et al., 2017). The ultimate goal of the standard is to identify "definitions and measurements of gender identity across the government to meet human rights requirements and to enable policy and service development for transgender [individuals]" (Pega et al., 2017, p. 219). New Zealand's initiation of the classification system will lead to improving health services and measurement of health outcomes for the country as well as place New Zealand as an international leader in transgender rights (Pega et al., 2017).

GERMANY

While Germany was a leader in transgender health dating back to the 18th century, most notably with physicians Harry Benjamin and Magnus Hirschfeld, the philosophy continues to pathologize gender nonconformity to allow for funding for gender confirming care (Nieder & Strauss, 2015). Additionally, Germany abides by the German Standards for the Treatment and Diagnostic Assessment of Transsexuals. Internationally, the WPATH Standards of Care are viewed as the pinnacle principles and ideals for treatment of the transgender population; the seventh revision was published in 2011 (Nieder & Strauss, 2015). However, the German standards have not been updated since the late 1990s (Nieder & Strauss, 2015), which has caused Germany to lag behind the rest of the modern world in caring for transgender individuals.

In response to the lack of updating to the German standards, Nieder and Strauss (2015) identify the need to improve access and care for transgender individuals. With this goal, Nieder and Strauss (2015) suggest the use of participatory approaches for transgender healthcare. Participatory approaches would utilize a patient-centered model providing care based on each individual's health needs along with instituting a collaborative relationship between the patient and healthcare provider (Nieder &

Strauss, 2015). This healthcare approach will improve patient autonomy, healthcare relationships, and informed decision making for transgender patients seeking care in Germany. Nieder and Strauss (2015) argue that participatory healthcare approaches will highlight evidence-based practice along with increasing the quality of Germany's provision of transgender-related care.

INDIA

In 2009, the Indian government began offering GCS for free to citizens, which is the only country in this region that provides this service, making India another leader in transgender healthcare (Balakrishnan, 2016). While not all transgender individuals may benefit from this service in India, the provision of this extensive and expensive surgery speaks volumes of the government and its stance on transgender rights. Additionally, Shaikh et al. (2016) identified the use of community-based organizations (CBOs) as a positive strategy to improve healthcare for the transgender population in India.

Shaikh et al's (2016) study identified how CBOs helped to improve access to care and connection to communities for transgender individuals in India. In this country, transgender individuals face barriers such as poverty, social and economic exclusion, and poor access to care due to their gender identity status (Shaikh et al., 2016). Project Pehchan is a 5-year program working at a national scale to fight AIDS, tuberculosis, and malaria. The Pehchan program, community-based programs that aim to educate and care for the transgender population, and attempts to improve access to a variety of services through CBOs for transgender individuals have as their main goal to increase empowerment among this population (Shaikh et al., 2016). With the use of pre- and post-intervention surveys, Shaikh et al. (2016) analyzed the outcomes of 268 transgender participants who took part in the services offered by the Pehchan program. Shaikh et al. (2016) found there was improved access to sexual and reproductive health services, HIV and STI education and testing, social support services, and higher confidence reported among the transgender participants in understanding their rights. Overall, the CBOs are offering a positive impact on the Indian transgender population. Despite these findings, Shaikh et al. (2016) recommend to decrease the incidence of minority stress among the transgender population that policies are legally enacted in the country in combination with the public services to further enhance health outcomes.

CANADA

Another leader in transgender healthcare is Canada, where the health coverage system funds GCS and other gender-related treatments for the gender minority populations (Balakrishnan, 2016). Additionally, Canadian medical programs are beginning to incorporate transgender health content into the curricula (Balakrishnan, 2016). Canada follows the WPATH Standards of Care when initiating and providing gender-related care to the transgender population, thereby ensuring mental healthcare is provided to all transgender individuals before pursuing GCS.

Toivonen and Dobson (2017) assessed the ethical issues that arise when performing psychosocial assessments for GCS for Canadian transgender clients. Based on the WPATH Standards of Care, Canadian surgeons who perform GCS require their transgender clients to have a diagnosis of gender dysphoria, HRT for 12 consecutive months, and a letter of recommendation written by the client's mental health provider (Toivonen & Dobson, 2017). With these requirements, Canadian mental health providers play a significant role and have great responsibility for the care of transgender clients seeking GCS.

Canadian mental health providers are responsible for upholding the four principles outlined in the *Canadian Code of Ethics for Psychologists.* Toivonen and Dobson (2017) describe how these four principles are applied to the transgender population. For instance, mental health providers should be aware of the autonomy of the client, understand the issues with long waiting lists for GCS in Canada, ensure reduction of harm, and maintain competency related to transgender healthcare (Toivonen & Dobson, 2017). Another important issue Canadian transgender individuals face is the lack of sites to receive GCS. Toivonen and Dobson (2017) identify only one "reputable and publicly funded" location for these services, which has an average waiting time of 7 months (2017, p. 180). This clinic is located in Quebec, which hinders those in other provinces with travel barriers the ability to access GCS. Therefore, despite the advances in policy and care Canada has to offer for the transgender population, there are major barriers to obtaining the care that is offered by health providers.

RURAL TRANSGENDER HEALTHCARE

Koch and Knutson (2016) provide an overview of the issues and barriers transgender individuals have accessing quality healthcare in rural settings.

While there are barriers for urban-dwelling transgender individuals, those who live in less populated, more conservative areas of the United States are impacted more due to the lack of support and available health services (Koch & Knutson, 2016). With issues such as transportation, lack of social and financial support, and biased or uninformed healthcare providers, rural transgender individuals may feel oppressed and marginalized to an extent urban transgender individuals may not experience. Additionally, the political and social climate of rural locations can create a large impact on the health services providers offer. Stigma, discrimination, and prejudice are issues transgender individuals face globally; however, when residing in an area of poor education, poverty, or conservative religious or political beliefs, the health experiences of transgender individuals are impacted.

Koch and Knutson (2016) offer recommendations based on the barriers identified in rural settings for transgender individuals. First, Koch and Knutson (2016) recommend establishing telehealth services to decrease the barrier related to transportation or distance. While this recommendation comes with its own barriers, such as lack of Internet or computer access, Koch and Knutson (2016) offer the recommendation of local libraries and health departments to provide video or telephone conference capabilities to allow access to telehealth services. Additionally, lack of social support can place barriers on transgender individuals, and Koch and Knutson (2016) recommend rural providers assist clients with connecting to LGBTQI groups or activities as well as identifying allies for clients who can help with managing relationships. While the issue of provider bias was not addressed by Koch and Knutson (2016), bias has been found to be a hindrance to receiving healthcare for many transgender individuals (Grant et al., 2011; James et al., 2016), and education on transgender needs and experiences can help to decrease the incidence of bias or prejudice from healthcare providers.

THE UNITED STATES

The United States has the most published research and literature on transgender health issues in the world (Reisner et al., 2016). While access to research and education has improved for U.S. healthcare providers, barriers and access to care are still limited for the transgender population due to social, historical, and political beliefs surrounding gender and gender expressions. With the institution of the Affordable Care Act in 2010, access and coverage for certain gender-related treatments improved;

however, coverage for GCS and access to HRT is still limited for many transgender individuals living in the United States today (Stroumsa, 2014).

Stroumsa (2014) identifies how the Affordable Care Act policy, through Medicare Part D, offers routine care and HRT for transgender individuals, but GCS is not covered. Additionally, not all states opted to include Part D when implementing the new healthcare bill, resulting in transgender individuals in those states not having coverage for HRT, if eligible for Medicare (Stroumsa, 2014). In response to the discrimination, violence, and lack of healthcare transgender individuals were experiencing, in May 2016, former president Obama initiated policies that ensured fair and equal treatment from all medical providers who receive Affordable Care Act funding (i.e., Medicaid and Medicare; Grubb, 2016). This policy protects transgender people from sex and gender discrimination in any federally funded institution, such as hospitals, clinics, or CBOs. However, only 19 states have laws or policies that prohibit private health insurers from excluding transgender health services (e.g., California, New York, Minnesota; National Center for Transgender Equality, 2016).

Another issue U.S. transgender individuals face includes the use of sex and gender interchangeably on health forms (Grubb, 2016). There are some institutions, agencies, and electronic health record providers that have implemented identifiers for sex assigned at birth, current gender identity or expression, and preferred pronoun; however, this is not seen consistently across the country (Grubb, 2016). For fair and standardized treatment of all clients of the healthcare system, it would be appropriate to institute these identifiers across all patient populations to become inclusive for transgender individuals.

One U.S. effort to improve transgender healthcare includes the U.S. Veterans Health Administration (VA) which aims to provide gender-related care in a standardized method to military veterans (Stroumsa, 2014). The transgender-related care the VA offers includes mental health, HRT, and preoperative and postoperative evaluation and care, but does not include GCS (Stroumsa, 2014). With the institution of these policies and provisions of medically necessary care, veterans receive more gender-related care than some U.S. civilians. The amount of progress seen in the VA in the last 6 years has led to an increase in transgender veterans' ability to access gender-related care. Additionally, the VA is dedicated to educate its employees in providing culturally sensitive care to transgender veterans (Stroumsa, 2014).

Similar to the initiatives of the VA, the Fenway Institute in Boston, MA, aims to provide extensive and inclusive care to the transgender population, along with sexual minorities (Reisner et al., 2015). Fenway Health is a comprehensive care environment that not only provides care to transgender individuals but also employs transgender individuals (Reisner et al., 2015). Thirty years ago, Fenway Health identified the issues transgender patients were having accessing care unrelated to HIV care, such as HRT and preventative care, and instituted a program to improve healthcare access for the Boston transgender community (Reisner et al., 2015). As part of Fenway Health, the Fenway Institute focuses on the care of the traditionally underserved. Through the Fenway Institute, education, advocacy, and research are at the forefront, and there have been collaborations globally to improve transgender healthcare (Reisner et al., 2015). Fenway Health also advocates for transgender rights and educates providers on how to provide care in an affirmative manner to transgender clients (Reisner et al., 2015).

THE FUTURE OF TRANSGENDER HEALTHCARE

While there are advocacy groups and health services available for transgender individuals, there are also widespread barriers, stigma, and discrimination (Grant et al., 2011; James et al., 2016), which coupled with the many global health systems that do not provide financial support for medically necessary therapies (i.e., HRT and GCS) can lead to negative mental and physical health outcomes for the transgender population (Stroumsa, 2014). Additionally, as the global population grows and gender fluidity and expression expands, research and healthcare will need to compensate for an aging transgender population and adolescents who opt for gender-related treatments at younger ages.

Additionally, health research continues to value heteronormative structures and practices when utilizing transgender participants in studies (Zeeman, Aranda, & Grant, 2014). For example, Zeeman et al. (2014) discuss how evidence-based research and practice aim to identify norms and exclusivity dependent on the population it is examining. However, in the realm of gender identity and expression, exclusion and normative roles are not appropriate nor is it fitting to demarcate gender nonconforming individuals to certain identities. Therefore, Zeeman et al. (2014) recommend researchers to be critical of the knowledge obtained in transgender studies and understand how power between healthcare, politics, society, and gender roles and expressions play a significant role in the transgender population due to the stigma and marginalization that is experienced.

Moreover, Merryfeather and Bruce (2014) identify the need for researchers to expand transgender health knowledge to understand the barriers to care as well as improve health outcomes for the marginalized population. And Reisner et al. (2016) stress the importance of identifying the number of transgender individuals globally in an effort to determine health needs and outcomes more effectively. With the growing awareness of transgender identities in the media, politics, and healthcare, the global health arena will need to place transgender issues on the forefront to improve access to quality and informed care for the community. Furthermore, the continued stigma and discrimination transgender individuals experience will continue to inflict issues upon this patient population both on mental and physical health. Therefore, it is not only healthcare that needs improvement but social and political thoughts will need to move in a positive and inclusive direction to minimize the effects this pronounced discrimination has had on transgender individuals and their health outcomes.

In summary, while visibility of the issues transgender individuals face is becoming more prominent in healthcare, particularly when assessing HIV risks and rates (Reisner et al., 2016), there continues to be invisibility to gender-related and preventative care for the transgender population. With select global initiatives, transgender patients are receiving better care than 30 years ago, yet many countries have not established policies or laws that protect transgender individuals from widespread discrimination or improve access to healthcare, including adequate financial support. This widespread discrimination has led to an increase in poor global health outcomes as well as continued stigma related to gender-nonconforming identities and expressions.

REFERENCES

Balakrishnan, V. S. (2016). Growing recognition of transgender health. *Bulletin of the World Health Organization, 94*, 790–791. doi:10.2471/BLT.16.021116

Grant, J. M., Mottet, L. A., Tanis, J., Harrison, J., Herman, J. L., & Keisling, M. (2011). Injustice at every turn: A Report of the National Transgender Discrimination Survey, Executive Summary. Retrieved from http://www.thetaskforce.org/static_html/downloads/reports/reports/ntds_summary.pdf

Grubb, H. M. (2016). Marginalization of transgender identities: Implications for health equity. *Psychiatric Annals, 46*(6), 334–339. doi:10.3928/00485713-20160418-01

Güldenring, A. (2015). A critical view of transgender health care in Germany: Psychopathologizing gender identity—Symptom of "disordered" psychiatric/psychological diagnostics? *International Review of Psychiatry, 27*(5), 427–434. doi:10.3109/09540261.2015.1083948

Institute of Medicine. (2011). *The health of lesbian, gay, bisexual, and transgender people: Building a foundation for better understanding.* Washington, DC: National Academies Press.

James, S. E., Herman, J. L., Rankin, S., Keisling, M., Mottet, L., & Anafi, M. (2016). *The report of the 2015 U.S. transgender survey.* Washington, DC: National Center for Transgender Equality. Retrieved from http://www .transequality.org/sites/default/files/docs/usts/USTS%20Full%20Report%20 -%20FINAL%201.6.17.pdf

Koch, J. M., & Knutson, D. (2016). Transgender clients in rural areas and small towns. *Journal of Rural Mental Health, 40*(3–4), 154–163. doi:10.1037/ rmh0000056

Merryfeather, L., & Bruce, A. (2014). The invisibility of gender diversity: Understanding transgender and transsexuality in nursing literature. *Nursing Forum, 49*(2), 110–123. doi:10.1111/nuf.12061

National Center for Transgender Equality. (2016). Map: State health insurance rates. Retrieved from http://www.transequality.org/issues/resources/ map-state-health-insurance-rules

National Center for Transgender Equality. (2017). Issues: Health & HIV. Retrieved from http://www.transequality.org/issues/health-hiv

Nieder, T. O., & Strauss, B. (2015). Transgender health care in Germany: Participatory approaches and the development of a guideline. *International Review of Psychiatry, 27*(5), 416–426. doi:10.3109/09540261.2015.1074562

Pega, F., Reisner, S. L., Sell, R. L., & Veale, J. F. (2017). Transgender health: New Zealand's innovative statistical standard for gender identity. *American Journal of Public Health, 107*(2), 217–221. doi:10.2105/AJPH.2016.303465

Pega, F., & Veale, J. F. (2015). The case for the World Health Organization's commission on social determinants of health to address gender identity. *American Journal of Public Health, 105*(3), 58–62. doi:10.2105/AJPH.2014.302373

Reisner, S. L., Bradford, J., Hopwood, R., Gonzalez, A., Makadon, H., Todisco, D., . . . Mayer, K. (2015). Comprehensive transgender healthcare: The gender affirming clinical and public health model for Fenway Health. *Journal of Urban Health: Bulletin of the New York Academy of Medicine, 92*(3), 584–592. doi:10.1007/s11524-015-9947-2

Reisner, S. L., Poteat, T., Keatley, J., Cabral, M., Mothopeng, T., Dunham, E., . . . Baral, S. D. (2016). Global health burden and needs of transgender populations: A review. *Lancet, 388*, 412–436. doi:10.1016/S0140-6736(16)00684-X

Riggs, D. W., Ansara, G. Y., & Treharne, G. J. (2015). An evidence-based model for understanding the mental health experiences of transgender Australians. *Australian Psychologist, 50,* 32–39. doi:10.1111/ap.12088

Shaikh, S., Mburu, G., Arumugam, V., Mattipalli, N., Aher, A., Mehta, S., & Robertson, J. (2016). Empowering communities and strengthening systems to improve transgender health: Outcomes from the Pehchan programme in India. *Journal of the International AIDS Society, 19*(3 Suppl. 2), 20809. doi:10.7448/IAS.19.3.20809

Stroumsa, D. (2014). The state of transgender health care: Policy, law, and medical frameworks. *American Journal of Public Health, 104*(3), e31–e38. doi:10.2105/AJPH.2013.301789

Terrell, K. (2011). *Black and transgender: A double burden.* Retrieved from https://www.theroot.com/black-and-transgender-a-double-burden-1790866418

Thomas, R., Pega, F., Khosla, R., Verster, A., Hana, T., & Say, L. (2017). Ensuring an inclusive global health agenda for transgender people. *Bulletin of the World Health Organization, 95,* 154–156. doi:10.2471/BLT.16.183913

Toivonen, K. I., & Dobson, K. S. (2017). Ethical issues in psychosocial assessment for sex reassignment surgery in Canada. *Canadian Psychology, 58*(2), 178–186. doi:10.1037/cap0000087

World Professional Association for Transgender Health. (2011). Standards of care for the health of transsexual, transgender, and gender nonconforming people (7th version). Retrieved from https://s3.amazonaws.com/amo_hub_content/Association140/files/Standards%20of%20Care%20V7%20-%202011%20WPATH%20(2)(1).pdf

Zeeman, L., Aranda, K., & Grant, A. (2014). Queer challenges to evidence-based practice. *Nursing Inquiry, 21*(2), 101–111. doi:10.1111/nin.12039

Human Trafficking and Global Health Issues

Donna Sabella
Mary de Chesnay

Human trafficking, also referred to as modern-day slavery, is a universal phenomenon impacting not only the United States but every country in the world (de Baca & Sigmon, 2014). The 2017 Trafficking in Persons (TIP) Report provides an overview of the types of human trafficking occurring in 187 countries as well as each country's attempts to combat this crime against humanity (U.S. Department of State, 2017). Human trafficking has been acknowledged as one of the fastest growing criminal industries in the world and one of the most lucrative forms of criminal activity as well as a multibillion-dollar global criminal enterprise (Arlacchi, 2000; Bureau of Justice Assistance, 2015).

Whereas a drug can be used only once, human beings can be repeatedly exploited, thereby making the selling and buying of human beings an extremely profitable endeavor. Human trafficking can consist of a variety of forms including forced labor, bonded labor, debt bondage, involuntary domestic servitude, forced child labor, child soldiering, organ trafficking, and sex trafficking (U.S. Department of State, 2009). According to various figures and estimates, which many agree are questionable owing to the covert nature of human trafficking, approximately 600,000 to 800,000 victims are trafficked yearly across international borders worldwide (U.S. Department of State, 2006), with approximately 14,500 to 17,500 of them ending up trafficked into the United States (U.S. Department of State, 2004).

Aside from international trafficking, domestic trafficking exists whereby American nationals, mainly girls and women, are moved from town to town and/or across state lines where they are forced into sexual exploitation and/or domestic servitude (Konstantopoulos et al., 2013). According to a number of sources, of particular concern is the increase in the sex trafficking of domestic minors in this country. Those working in the healthcare field, especially nurses, and in the human services fields, including social workers and psychologists, and those involved in the criminal justice field need to be aware of what trafficking is, the extent to which trafficking occurs, and how to identify, support, and treat trafficking victims. The odds are likely that at some point we will come across trafficking victims, many of whom are often hidden right in front of us in plain sight.

While sex trafficking is the form of human trafficking most highlighted in the news and the form of trafficking more commonly recognized by the public, it is not the only type of trafficking that exists. Typically, this phenomenon is divided into two broad categories: sex trafficking and labor trafficking. Definitions of trafficking vary depending on who is defining it, but a common description often used for all forms of human trafficking includes the criteria of force, fraud, and coercion as means of recruiting and controlling victims (U.S. Congress, 2000; U.S. Department of Health and Human Services, 2012). Sex trafficking involves the exploitation of an individual for the purposes of providing sexual services against their will. Among other places, victims can commonly be found working in brothels, massage parlors, hotels, casinos, on the streets, and through escort services.

Labor trafficking involves exploiting individuals to work against their will often through force, fraud, or coercion (U.S. Congress, 2000; U.S. Department of Health and Human Services, 2012). Among other places, victims can be found working in factories, farms, hotels, restaurants, nail salons, or private homes as domestic servants.

Two lesser known manifestations of human trafficking are organ trafficking and sex tourism. Organ trafficking involves the involuntary removal of human organs from an individual for the purpose of transplantation (Capron & Delmonico, 2015; Jafar, 2009). In the United States, selling an organ for profit is illegal, but there are other countries where it is legal. The key difference is that the individual agrees to donate an organ and can expect to be appropriately reimbursed.

Finally, sex tourism typically consists of men traveling to other countries where they have arranged tours that enable them to have sex with individuals in that country. While the tour can include having sex with adults, the tours are often designed to provide access to children with whom the men have sex (Bales & Soodalter, 2009; de Chesnay, 2012).

Healthcare professionals are well situated to come into contact with human trafficking victims and survivors in a number of contexts and situations. While historically not part of most nursing programs' curricula at either the undergraduate or graduate levels, nursing is becoming more aware of this phenomenon and a number of schools have begun offering some training or coursework to students in addition to including presentations on human trafficking at numerous nursing conferences. It is important that nurses become knowledgeable about this topic, including how to recognize possible signs and symptoms of human trafficking. It is also critical for nurses to become familiar with human trafficking policies both here and abroad. Toward that end, the chapter begins with a literature review followed by a discussion of health issues common in and related to human trafficking, and a discussion of human trafficking health-related policies both in the United States and abroad. The chapter concludes with thoughts related to what does and does not work and an overview of future recommendations.

POLICY LITERATURE REVIEW

In recent years, researchers have focused attention on issues related to human trafficking as the phenomenon becomes more visible to the general public. The following section highlights the policy literature related to human trafficking and can be categorized into several discrete focus areas: controversy over linking abortion politics with the Trafficking Victims Protection Act (TVPA); anti-trafficking policies and laws; economic migration; and protection of children.

ABORTION POLITICS

Having sailed to reauthorization in previous years with great consensus in Congress, the 2011 TVPA ran into partisan opposition from antiabortion groups because the Department of Health and Human Services did not renew funds to Catholic organizations that refused to provide abortion and contraceptive services to victims. By making the TVPA a "women's issue," the antiabortion resistance distracted the attention of Congress to the real crux of human trafficking—that it is a male and female issue.

The author suggests that in the future, lawmakers focus on both forced labor and sex trafficking (Bewley, 2014).

ANTI-TRAFFICKING POLICIES AND LAWS

In the United States, the primary law protecting trafficking victims is the TVPA, first authorized in 2000 and renewed several times since. The TVPA originally provided protection to victims of trafficking and domestic violence. Subsequent reauthorizations expanded protections and services to victims and mandated penalties for traffickers. The TVPA also recognized the issues specific to refugees and persons trafficked across borders and makes provision for victims trafficked to the United States from other countries (U.S. Department of State, 2000).

ECONOMIC MIGRATION

Human trafficking is a natural consequence of economic migration from poor countries. Individuals move for a variety of reasons but mostly having to do with improving their families' safety and economic well-being (Mahmoud & Trebesch, 2010). If mass migration increases human trafficking risk, then it seems logical to say that individuals are at greater risk by moving away from their homes and support systems to new countries where they are strangers without support systems to protect and guide them. Traffickers are adept at convincing vulnerable individuals that they will protect them and thereby place them in states of extreme subservience and dependence.

PROTECTION OF CHILDREN

Children are among the most vulnerable not only to the traffickers but also to their own families. Desperate people do bad things and parents who cannot feed their large families sell some of their children into slavery by convincing themselves they are doing the best they can for their families as a whole. Not only do traffickers make promises to protect, feed, and educate the children but they might also pay the families a sum to let the child go.

In the United States, legislation has targeted child sex trafficking. The Preventing Sex Trafficking and Strengthening Families Act, P.L. 113-183, was signed into law in September 2014 (www.congress.gov/bill/113th-congress/house-bill/4980/text). The act requires Title IV-E agencies to develop ways to identify and provide services for children in foster care at risk for being targeted for the sex trade (Child Welfare and Human Trafficking Brief, 2017).

GLOBAL ANTI-TRAFFICKING POLICIES

The Department of State publishes the annual TIP Report that includes rankings and examples from many countries of human trafficking. In the 2016 report, special attention was given to the vulnerability of populations from regions of armed conflict, protracted crises, and natural disasters (U.S. Department of State, 2016). Continued attention is given to the governments of Syria, Iraq, Libya, Haiti, Nepal, the Philippines, eastern and northern Africa, Yemen, and tsunami-affected areas of Indonesia, Sri Lanka, and Thailand. Poverty, hopelessness, lack of education, and corruption exploit vulnerability for the profit of the few at the expense of the many.

HEALTH ISSUES RELATED TO HUMAN TRAFFICKING

Human beings who are trafficked do not present with a sign or label stating as much. In fact, while they may reveal other things about themselves, at times they may be reluctant to share that they are being exploited, and in some cases, they may not realize that they are being victimized. In an emergency department, a woman complaining of shortness of breath, provocatively dressed, with the word "Daddy" tattooed on her neck, and numerous unopened condom wrappers and hand sanitizer in her handbag brought in by two men who do not let her speak may be easily recognized as a possible victim. However, that is not always the case and nurses need to be aware of more subtle signs and clues that could indicate possible victimization. A good start involves understanding some of the common health issues related to human trafficking. It is important to remember that not all individuals will present with the following conditions, and that some individuals are trafficked with any number of preexisting conditions. Victims, whether sex or labor trafficked, typically suffer from a variety of problems stemming from, among other things, inhumane and unsanitary living arrangements, poor personal hygiene, poor nutrition, dangerous and unhealthy working conditions, physical and emotional abuse, and, of course, a lack of consistent and quality healthcare.

Also, it is important to remember that in and of itself, a given health problem or issue does not necessarily mean someone is being trafficked. Plenty of non-trafficked individuals suffer from the same medical, emotional, and physical problems as those who are trafficked. Rather, each piece of information about the individual, including non-health factors, is a piece of the puzzle that needs to have at least most, if not all, pieces in place before the whole picture becomes visible. Typically, while they share much in common, health issues can be considered from a sex trafficking or labor trafficking perspective.

SEX TRAFFICKING

Just as is the case with non-victims, human trafficking victims can present with a variety of health problems, not all of which are typically thought of as being related to sexual activity. These would include any number of undetected or untreated diseases, such as diabetes, cancer, or respiratory infections, including pneumonia and bronchitis, or any number of cardiovascular-related health problems. However, there are also a number of health and medical problems presented below which tend to be related to sexual exploitation (Acharya & Clark, 2010; de Chesnay & Greenbaum, 2013; Dovydaitis, 2010; Lederer & Wetzel, 2014; Oram, Stöckl, Busza, Howard, & Zimmerman, 2012; Richards, 2014; Sabella, 2011, 2013, 2015; Taylor & Blake, 2013; Zimmerman, 2006; Zimmerman, Hossain, & Watts, 2011):

- Genital problems, including signs of sexual assault: vaginal and rectal tears, fistulas, abrasions, swelling, and lacerations

- Unwanted or unplanned pregnancies and/or signs of multiple abortions

- HIV and/or AIDS

- Amenorrhea or menstrual abnormalities

- Frequent urinary tract as well as sexually transmitted infections: trichomoniasis; hepatitis A, B, and C; syphilis; gonorrhea; human papillomavirus (HPV); genital herpes; and chlamydia

- Pelvic inflammatory disease (PID)

- Various physical injuries indicating assault and physical abuse: missing teeth, broken bones, sprains and bruises, stab wounds, gunshot wounds, bite marks, burns, black eyes, pulled hair

- Temporal mandibular joint disease

- Dermatological problems: track marks, scabies, rashes, and various skin infections

- Tattoos or brandings

- Headaches

- Backaches

- Hearing loss

- Dental problems including missing teeth

- Substance use disorders and/or addiction

- Gastrointestinal problems along with eating disorders and poor nutrition

- Numerous psychological issues including psychological trauma, depression, stress-related disorders, anxiety, disorientation, confusion, phobias, panic attacks, PTSD, and suicidal ideation

LABOR TRAFFICKING

Similar to sex trafficking victims, labor trafficking victims can present with any number of health problems, including those unrelated to being exploited for labor trafficking. However, as is the case with those exploited for sex trafficking, there are a number of medical and health problems provided below which are commonly associated with labor trafficking victimization (Napolitano, 2016; Rescue and Restore, n.d.; U.S. Department of Health and Human Services, 2012):

- Chronic back, hearing, cardiovascular or respiratory problems from endless days working in dangerous agriculture, sweatshop, or construction conditions and being exposed to hazardous materials

- Loss of limbs, fingers, or toes owing to working with machinery

- Signs of intentional disfigurement including being blinded

- Signs of physical abuse such as scars, broken bones

- Weak eyes and other eye and vision problems from working in dimly lit sweatshops

- Malnourishment, dehydration, and failure to thrive

- Serious dental problems

- Infectious diseases like tuberculosis

- Undetected or untreated diseases, such as diabetes or cancer

- Bruises, scars, and other signs of physical abuse and torture

- Poor personal hygiene

- Hyperthermia or hypothermia

- Psychological symptoms including anxiety, depression, PTSD, and suicidal ideation

ORGAN TRAFFICKING

Aside from the two major categories of human trafficking, we need to consider victims of organ trafficking. While selling organs is against the law in the United States, in other countries it is permitted. While some argue in favor of allowing individuals to decide to sell an organ for profit, others express concern that in some cases what might appear at first glance as the individual freely agreeing and wishing to do so could, on closer inspection, reveal some measure of the individual agreeing to do so for questionable reasons (Capron & Delmonico, 2015). A clear sign that someone is the victim of organ harvesting would be surgical incisions or scars.

WHAT WORKS: WHAT DOESN'T WORK

Those exploited for whatever type of trafficking will, in all likelihood, develop some sort of health problems during their victimization in addition to what other health problems they may bring with them at the time of their exploitation. Preexisting medical and behavioral conditions can be expected to worsen, not improve, during the period in which individuals are being exploited and trafficked. For many human trafficking victims, access to healthcare and treatment prior to their victimization may have been limited or nonexistent—a situation which continues to be the case during their victimization. Victims receive no healthcare benefits, and while some may receive adequate care, depending on their situation, it is not unusual for victims to suffer from lack of care, or from receiving substandard care.

While policies can provide guidance and opportunities for victims to receive the healthcare they need, they could still fall between the cracks and not receive that care if they are not accurately identified by health-care providers. It is therefore imperative that any policy related to the healthcare needs of human trafficking individuals also address the need to properly train healthcare providers regarding the fundamentals of what human trafficking is, how to identify and support victims, and how to make proper referrals for them. As healthcare providers, we would expect that they already know how to treat the various medical and behavioral conditions and issues that victims present with. But before that treatment can begin, healthcare providers, including nurses, need to know what human trafficking is and how to properly identify possible victims.

Aside from the above importance of being able to correctly identify and treat possible human trafficking victims, it is important to view the phenomenon of human trafficking on a larger scale. Todres (2011a) suggests widening our lens in terms of how society views human trafficking. He points out that viewing human trafficking from a criminal law perspective has proved rather fruitless in combating human trafficking and reducing its incidence (Todres, 2011b). He cites the United States' historically three-pronged approach in dealing with human trafficking as requiring punishing perpetrators, protecting and providing assistance to victims, and developing prevention measures (Todres, 2011b). Yet, unfortunately, as he points out, while most efforts universally have tended toward criminal law efforts and policies to combat the problem, little has been done to help victims and to develop programs whose focus is on prevention. Especially concerning is that in the end criminal law and its various related policies do little to address and improve the health of those who have been trafficked or to provide victim assistance or prevent human trafficking (Todres, 2011b).

As detailed in the above section on health issues related to human trafficking, we know that victims can experience a wide range of physical, emotional, and/or sexual abuses from a variety of those with whom they come in contact, including not just traffickers or pimps, but from employers, clients, and at times, even their own family members, as we read of reports about honor killings and banishment of victims by their families and cases where victims are intentionally forced into labor or sex trafficking by their own family members. The consequences on victims' health can be long lasting and even life-threatening.

A PUBLIC HEALTH PERSPECTIVE

So, what, we may ask, can be done to improve the situation in terms of human trafficking and global health issues? We can begin with what we know, which is that human trafficking–related abuses create and worsen a wide variety of medical, physical, and behavioral diseases, illnesses, and disorders among those who have been victimized (Neupane & Kallestrup, 2015; Zimmerman, Hossain, & Watts, 2011). We can move away from considering human trafficking solely or largely through a lens of crime and punishment, and include other perspectives such as a development or human rights perspective (Todres, 2011a). A rallying call offered several years back and seeming to gain more momentum at present is to view human trafficking as a public health issue (Chisolm-Straker & Stoklosa, 2017; Relentless, 2013; Todres, 2011a, 2011b; U.S. Department of Health and Human Services, 2016; Welch, 2013; Zimmerman, Hossain, & Watts, 2011).

While beyond the scope of this chapter to fully address the merits of such an approach and perspective, the argument can be made that human trafficking impacts large numbers of people worldwide, and as such has population-level implications and consequences, both present and future. In addition, human trafficking creates numerous health problems for human trafficking victims, some of which are severe and long lasting. Many of these are already considered public health issues—such as violence, communicable and noncommunicable diseases, and addiction, all of which add to the global health burden (Welch, 2013). Public health places heavy emphasis on prevention, an area that needs more focus, attention, and action in the fight against human trafficking—and evidence-based research, another area sorely needed (Todres, 2011b; Welch, 2013). In addition, public health is known for developing appropriate treatment guidelines and evaluating healthcare outcomes—again, an area lacking in our current efforts to combat human trafficking (Todres, 2011b; Welch, 2013). Our efforts to this phenomenon need to be more proactive and less reactive.

FUTURE RECOMMENDATIONS

So where do we go from here as we move toward the future? We are now many years into our awareness of human trafficking. Almost two decades ago, the United States created and passed the TVPA of 2000, with various reauthorizations of this initial federal law enacted in the ensuing years. In addition, the United States went on to establish the yearly TIP Report, available every June online, which provides information about the types of trafficking occurring in countries included in the report and their efforts to combat human trafficking. Yet there is still more to be done, especially related to healthcare and healthcare professionals. As de Baca and Sigmon (2014) point out, human trafficking continues to remain a hidden crime and presents a fundamental challenge in terms of identifying victims and offering appropriate services to them, particularly healthcare services. They, as well as others, call for the development and implementation of educational courses and training programs for healthcare professionals to improve the recognition of human trafficking victims and provision of services to victims (Ahn et al., 2013; de Baca & Sigmon, 2014; Goldenberg, 2015; Isaac, Solak, & Giardino, 2011).

In a recent study on the state of affairs regarding required training and education, Atkinson, Curnin, and Hanson (2016) report that 17 states have enacted legislation that either specifically addresses the education of healthcare providers and other professionals about human trafficking (13 states), requires mandatory reporting of trafficking of minors (seven states), or compels both (three states) (p. 114). Clearly this is not the majority of states. In terms of nursing professionals, an informal survey of required continuing education courses that focused specifically on human trafficking revealed that no states required such education for nursing licensure renewal (Sabella & McCain Institute, 2017). Likewise, a similar state of affairs exists when examining the content and curriculum of both undergraduate and graduate nursing programs in the United States. Only a few offer any training about human trafficking, and those that do tend to offer it as an elective. In fact, several schools declined an offer by one of the authors to develop and teach a course about human trafficking.

It is, at this stage, premature to declare what works as we are still searching for answers to what is a question, not a statement. However, with that caveat in mind, the following are but a few suggestions that have been put forth as reasonable possibilities for improving the identification and treatment of human trafficking victims by healthcare professionals, including nurses (American Public Health Association, 2015; de Baca & Sigmon, 2014;

Macy & Graham, 2012; World Health Organization, 2012; Zimmerman & Borland, 2009; Zimmerman, Hossain, & Watts, 2011):

- Develop and implement new training and education programs for healthcare professionals at all levels; the education should include information about the contexts in which trafficking presently exists

- Develop international and global connections among healthcare providers to share information about human trafficking, including challenges and advances

- Integrate human trafficking into existing curricula on domestic violence, intimate partner violence, and child and elder abuse

- Draw on interventions that have proven effective with other similarly vulnerable populations—such as torture survivors, domestic abuse victims, and migrant laborers

- Increase government involvement and spending on research related to physical and mental consequences of being trafficked

- Use federal, state, and private resources to evaluate health provider human trafficking training and prevention programs

- Work to develop trauma-informed policies and procedures that are also linguistically and culturally appropriate and sensitive to meeting the medical and behavioral needs of victims

- Involve survivors' input in both program development and evaluation outcome

- Enact goverment-mandated acute and long-term provision of healthcare to human trafficking victims

- Gather more empirical data on the healthcare needs of trafficked men

While it is safe to say that efforts to improve the health and healthcare services provided to victims of human trafficking should be considered works in progress, they also, as the saying goes, should be considered a journey of a thousand miles beginning with the first step. Hopefully, the above recommendations provide suggestions for not just first steps in this journey but steps in the right direction.

SUMMARY

This chapter has reviewed several policy issues related to human trafficking, with particular attention to the health issues of sex trafficking survivors and needed reforms in the way services are provided. Human trafficking in all its forms is a global health problem. Although progress has been made in calling attention to the extent and severity of human trafficking, more progress on reducing demand for trafficked persons and improving services to victims/survivors is needed if we are to reverse the course of what might be called a pandemic.

REFERENCES

Acharya, A. K., & Clark, J. B. (2010). The health consequences of trafficking in women in Mexico: Findings from Monterrey City. *International Review of Sociology, 20*(3), 415–426. doi:10.1080/03906701.2010.511886

Ahn, R., Albert, E., Purcell, G., Konstantopoulos, W., McGahan, A., Cafferty, E., ... Burke, T. (2013). Human trafficking: review of educational resources for health professionals. *American Journal of Preventive Medicine, 44*(3), 283–289. doi:10.1016/j.amepre.2012.10.025

American Public Health Association. (2015). Expanding and coordinating human trafficking-related public health research, evaluation, education, and prevention (Policy Number 201516). Retrieved from https://www.apha.org/policies-and -advocacy/public-health-policy-statements/policy-database/2016/01/26/14/28/ expanding-and-coordinating-human-trafficking-related-public-health-activities

Arlacchi, P. (2000). *International seminar on trafficking in human beings.* Vienna, Austria: United Nations Office on Drugs and Crime. Retrieved from http:// www.unodc.org/unodc/en/about-unodc/speeches/speech_2000-11-28_1.html

Atkinson, H. G., Curnin, K. J., & Hanson, N. C. (2016). U.S. state laws addressing human trafficking: Education of and mandatory reporting by health care providers and other professionals. *Journal of Human Trafficking, 2*(2), 111–138. doi:10.1080/23322705.2016.1175885

Bales K., & Soodalter, R. (2009). Supply and demand. In *The slave next door: Human trafficking and slavery in America today* (pp. 78–116). Berkeley: University of California Press.

Bewley, E. (2014). A new form of "Ideological Capture": Abortion politics and the Human Trafficking Protection Act. *Harvard Law & Policy Review, 8*(1), 229–253. Retrieved from http://harvardlpr.com/wp-content/uploads/2014/03/Bewley.pdf

Bureau of Justice Assistance, U.S. Department of Justice. (2015). Anti-human trafficking task force initiative: Overview. Retrieved from https://www.bja .gov/ProgramDetails.aspx?Program_ID=51

Capron, A. M., & Delmonico, F. L. (2015). Preventing trafficking in organs for transplantation: An important facet of the fight against human trafficking. *Journal of Human Trafficking, 1*(1), 56–64. doi:10.1080/23322705.2015.1011491

Child Welfare and Human Trafficking Brief. (2017). Author. Retrieved from https://www.childwelfare.gov/pubPDFs/trafficking_caseworkers.pdf

Chisolm-Straker, M., & Stoklosa, H. (Eds.). (2017). *Human trafficking is a public health issue: A paradigm expansion in the United States.* Cham, Switzerland: Springer.

de Baca, L. C., & Sigmon, J. N. (2014). Combating trafficking in persons: A call to action for global health professionals. *Global Health: Science and Practice, 2*(3), 261–267. doi:10.9745/GHSP-D-13-00142. Retrieved from http://www .ghspjournal.org/content/2/3/261.full.pdf+html

de Chesnay, M. (2012). Sex trafficking and sex tourism. In M. de Chesnay & B. Anderson (Eds.), *Caring for the vulnerable: Perspectives in nursing theory, practice and research* (pp. 385–392). Sudbury, MA: Jones and Bartlett.

de Chesnay, M., & Greenbaum, J. (2013). Physical trauma. In M. de Chesnay (Ed.), *Sex trafficking: A clinical guide for nursing* (pp. 263–280). New York, NY: Springer Publishing.

Dovydaitis, T. (2010). Human trafficking: The role of the healthcare provider. *Journal of Midwifery and Women's Health, 55*(5), 462–467. doi:10.1016/ j.jmwh.2009.12.017

Goldenberg, S. M. (2015). Trafficking, migration, and health: Complexities and future directions. *The Lancet Global Health, 3*(3), e118–e119. doi:10.1016/ S2214-109X(15)70082-3. Retrieved from http://www.thelancet.com/journals/ langlo/article/PIIS2214-109X(15)70082-3/fulltext.

Isaac, R., Solak, J., & Giardino, A. (2011). Health care providers' training needs related to human trafficking: Maximizing the opportunity to effectively screen and intervene. *Journal of Applied Research on Children, 2*(1), Article 8. Retrieved from http://digitalcommons.library.tmc.edu/childrenatrisk/vol2/iss1/8

Jafar, T. H. (2009). Organ trafficking: Global solutions for a global problem. *American Journal of Kidney Diseases, 54*(6), 1145–1157. doi:10.1053/ j.ajkd.2009.08.014

Konstantopoulos, W. M., Ahn, R., Alpert, E. J., Cafferty, E., McGahan, A., Williams, T. P., ... Burke, T. F. (2013). An international comparative public health analysis of sex trafficking of women and girls in eight cities: Achieving a more effective health sector response. *Journal of Urban Health: Bulletin of the New York Academy of Medicine, 90*(6), 1194–1204. doi:10.1007/s11524-013-9837-4

Lederer, L. J., & Wetzel C. A. (2014). The health consequences of sex trafficking and their implications for identifying victims in healthcare facilities. *Annals of Health Law, 23*(1), 61–91. Retrieved from http://www.globalcenturion.org/ wp-content/uploads/2014/08/The-Health-Consequences-of-Sex-Trafficking.pdf

Macy, R., & Graham, L. (2012). Identifying domestic and international sex-trafficking victims during human service provision. *Trauma, Violence, & Abuse 13*(2), 59–76. doi:10.1177/1524838012440340

Mahmoud, T., & Trebesch, C. (2010). The economics of human trafficking and labour migration: Micro-evidence from Europe. Retrieved from http://conference .iza.org/conference_files/LeIlli2010/trebesch_c4269.pdf

Napolitano, K. (2016). *Human trafficking: A public health issue.* Retrieved from http://combathumantrafficking.org/2016/12/human-trafficking-a-public -health-issue

Neupane, D., & Kallestrup, A. (2015). *Human trafficking: An emerging global health problem.* Retrieved from http://www.globalhealthminders.dk/wp -content/uploads/2015/01/GHM-HumanTrafficking-Brief.pdf

Oram S., Stöckl, H., Busza, J., Howard, L. M., & Zimmerman, C. (2012). Prevalence and risk of violence and the physical, mental, and sexual health problems associated with human trafficking: Systematic review. *PLoS Medicine, 9*(5), e1001224. doi:10.1371/journal.pmed.1001224. Retrieved from http:// journals.plos.org/plosmedicine/article?id=10.1371/journal.pmed.1001224

Relentless. (2013). *Human trafficking IS a public health issue.* Retrieved from https://gorelentless.wordpress.com/2013/05/01/human-trafficking-is-a -public-health-issue

Rescue and Restore. (n.d.). *Common health issues seen in victims of human trafficking.* Retrieved from https://www.acf.hhs.gov/sites/default/files/orr/ health_problems_seen_in_traffick_victims.pdf

Richards, T. A. (2014). Health implications of human trafficking. *Nursing for Women's Health, 18*(2), 155–162. doi:10.1111/1751-486X.12112

Sabella, D. (2011). The role of the nurse in combating human trafficking. *American Journal of Nursing, 111*(2), 28–37. doi:10.1097/01.NAJ.0000394289.55577.b6

Sabella, D. (2013). Health issues and interactions with adult survivors. In M. de Chesnay (Ed.), *Sex trafficking: A clinical guide for nurses* (pp. 483–518). New York, NY: Springer Publishing Company.

Sabella, D. (2015). Emerging issues: Human trafficking. In B. Price & K. Maguire (Eds.), *Core curriculum for forensic nursing* (pp. 200–220). New York, NY: Wolters Kluwer.

Sabella, D., & The McCain Institute. (2017). *Informal survey of U.S. State Boards of Nursing and their human trafficking requirement for CE credits.* Unpublished by authors.

Taylor, G., & Blake, B. (2013). Sexually transmitted infections. In M. de Chesnay (Ed.), *Sex trafficking: A clinical guide for nurses* (pp. 239–262). New York, NY: Springer Publishing Company.

Todres, J. (2011a). Widening our lens: Incorporating essential perspectives in the fight against human trafficking. *Michigan Journal of International Law, 33*(1), 53–76. Georgia State University College of Law, Legal Studies Research Paper No. 2011-29. Retrieved from SSRN: https://ssrn.com/abstract=1958164

Todres, J. (2011b). Moving upstream: The merits of a public health law approach to human trafficking. *North Carolina Law Review, 89*(2), 447–506. Georgia State University College of Law, Legal Studies Research Paper No. 2011-02. Retrieved from SSRN: https://ssrn.com/abstract=1742953

U.S. Congress. (2000). *Victims of Trafficking and Violence Protection Act of 2000.* Public Law 106-386. Retrieved from https://www.state.gov/documents/organization/10492.pdf

U.S. Department of Health and Human Services. (2012). *Fact sheet: Human trafficking.* Washington, DC: Author. Retrieved from https://www.acf.hhs.gov/otip/resource/fact-sheet-human-trafficking

U.S. Department of Health and Human Services. (2016). The power of framing human trafficking as a public health issue. Retrieved from https://www.acf.hhs.gov/otip/resource/publichealthlens

U.S. Department of State. (2000). *Victims of Trafficking and Violence Protection Act of 2000.* Washington, DC: Author. Retrieved from https://www.state.gov/j/tip/laws/61124.htm

U.S. Department of State. (2004). *Trafficking in persons report 2006*. Washington, DC: Author. Retrieved from https://www.state.gov/j/tip/rls/tiprpt/2004

U.S. Department of State. (2006). *Trafficking in persons report 2006*. Washington, DC: Author. Retrieved from https://www.state.gov/g/tip/rls/tiprpt/2006/

U.S. Department of State. (2009). *Trafficking in persons report 2009*. Washington, DC: Author. Retrieved from https://www.state.gov/j/tip/rls/tiprpt/2009/

U.S. Department of State. (2016). *Trafficking in persons report 2016*. Washington, DC: Author. Retrieved from https://www.state.gov/j/tip/rls/tiprpt/2016/

U.S. Department of State. (2017). *Trafficking in persons report 2017*. Washington, DC: Author. Retrieved from https://www.state.gov/j/tip/rls/tiprpt/2017/

Welch, K. (2013). Human trafficking is a public health problem. Retrieved from https://cancerincytes.scienceblog.com/2013/02/21/human-trafficking-is-a-public-health-problem/

World Health Organization. (2012). Human Trafficking. Retrieved from http://apps.who.int/iris/bitstream/10665/77394/1/WHO_RHR_12.42_eng.pdf

Zimmerman, C. (2006). The health risks and consequences of trafficking in women and adolescents: Findings from a European study. *London School of Hygiene and Tropical Medicine*. Retrieved from http://www.lshtm.ac.uk/hpu/docs/traffickingfinal.pdf.

Zimmerman, C., & Borland, R. (Eds.) (2009). *Caring for trafficked persons: Guidance for health providers*. Geneva, Switzerland: International Organization for Migration. Retrieved from http://publications.iom.int/system/files/pdf/ct_handbook.pdf

Zimmerman, C., Hossain, M., & Watts, C. (2011). Human trafficking and health: A conceptual model to inform policy, intervention and research. *Social Science & Medicine, 73*(2), 327–335. doi:10.1016/j.socscimed.2011.05.028

Global Trends in Criminalizing HIV Nondisclosure: Implications for Nursing Practice

Jennifer M. Kilty
Evelina W. Sterling
Portia D. Thomas

Time is both a gift and a curse. In terms of the initial political and public health responses to HIV in the early 1980s, an era of panic and uncertainty, it was a curse. Fear and ignorance generated stigma associated with HIV and by extension, people living with HIV/AIDS (PLWHA). HIV transmission was thought to be exclusive to marginalized groups that were assumed to be deviant and immoral—notably gay men, intravenous drug users, sex workers, and Haitian immigrants. The gift of time has also allowed science to produce epidemiological evidence of HIV's progression based on risk behaviors rather than identity characteristics. Despite significant scientific advancement in the treatment of HIV making it a chronic manageable condition instead of a death sentence, public misconception about the risk of transmission and stigma remains.

A growing global trend in criminalizing HIV nondisclosure demonstrates that public knowledge about HIV has not evolved with time. In general, HIV criminalization describes the unjust application of the criminal law to PLWHA based solely on their HIV status. This can include HIV-specific criminal statutes or applying existing criminal laws that allow for the prosecution of unintentional HIV transmission, potential or perceived exposure to HIV where HIV was not transmitted, and nondisclosure of known HIV-positive status. HIV criminalization laws emerged in the United States in 1986 (Lazzarini et al., 2013; Lehman et al., 2014). To ensure compliance, HIV federal funding was tied to policies pertaining to HIV disclosure. For instance, the 1990 Ryan White Comprehensive AIDS Resources Emergency (CARE) Act required states to confirm that they have the capability to prosecute PLWHA for deliberate exposure (Centers for Disease Control and Prevention [CDC], 2015b).

Criminalization is not based on scientific or medical evidence, but rather fear and a lack of knowledge about the risks of transmission and the efficiency of modern antiretroviral treatment (Csete & Elliott, 2011). In fact, a recent study found no association between HIV or AIDS diagnosis rates and criminal exposure laws across U.S. states over time, suggesting that these laws have had no detectable HIV prevention effect (Sweeney et al., 2017). Consequently, criminalization creates injustice and discrimination against PLWHA and is best considered an extrapunitive juridical measure. Still, the Joint United Nations Programme on HIV/AIDS (UNAIDS, 2010) reports that 56 countries have laws that specifically criminalize HIV transmission and exposure while other countries, like Canada, use existing criminal code legislation to criminalize nondisclosure. Critically examining the outcomes of the criminalization of HIV nondisclosure is required not only by governmental agencies but also by healthcare and nursing professionals working on the frontlines of HIV/AIDS care. Considering the ways in which criminalization is incongruent with evolving medical knowledge, efforts to achieve universal access to HIV prevention, treatment, care, and support are critical.

Due to the initial lack of knowledge regarding modes and risks of transmission and the fatality of the illness at the time, a distinction made between HIV and other sexually transmitted infections (STIs) was appropriate in the 1980s. Given the evolution of our scientific knowledge about HIV and the fact that advancements in treatment have made the illness a chronic but manageable condition, this severe distinction is no longer considered medically necessary. HIV is an STI, which means that its modes of transmission are the same as other STIs, including syphilis, genital herpes, gonorrhea, and chlamydia; problematically however, these STIs are not perceived with the same level of fear and stigma. The main argument in support of continuing to mark HIV/AIDS as exceptional arises in relation to the potentiality for mortality, despite the fact that similar risks exist with other untreated STIs. Moreover, people who contract STIs are at an increased risk of contracting HIV. The application of criminal law to HIV increases stigma and discrimination against PLWHA, thus driving them further away from appropriate HIV prevention, treatment, care, and support services.

The criminalization of HIV nondisclosure does not reflect the advancement of current medical science. Antiretroviral therapy has been a spectacular success, and with early diagnosis and treatment PLWHA can live nearly as long as seronegative people (Deeks, Lewin, & Havlir, 2013). Still, erroneous information and misconceptions about HIV persist. For example, fear and ignorance lead many people to believe that any bodily fluids are avenues for transmission. As a result, some HIV-specific laws criminalize exposure via spitting and biting (Center for HIV Law and Policy [CHLP], 2015; Jurgens et al., 2009; Lehman et al., 2014), which is not only unfair to PLWHA but is also misleading to the public as the courts are propagating misinformation about the risks and vectors of transmission.

Because nurses are on the frontlines of healthcare provision and educational awareness for PLWHA, criminalization negatively impacts this relationship by threatening patient trust and confidentiality when case notes may be subpoenaed in a criminal trial and healthcare practitioners may be called to testify in court (Sanders 2014). O'Bryne (2011) and Jurgens et al. (2009) suggest that nurses should recognize the impact of these laws and advocate for patients by educating and documenting that PLWHA and screened patients were counseled on criminalization. For nurses and other healthcare providers, documentation provides legal protection for their practice, licenses, and institutions, but it may create unintended consequences for PLWHA.

Nurses have been found to disagree with informing patients of the legal ramifications of nondisclosure, which was considered to be an unreasonable burden that diverts their focus away from HIV care and counseling (Sanders, 2014). Nurses struggle between deciding if they will provide information on criminalization, withhold this information, or provide it upon request (Sanders, 2014). Additionally, possible media coverage can breech anonymity locally, nationally, and even globally (Kilty, 2014; Shevory, 2004). Although unknown currently, nurses and healthcare providers might eventually be responsible for reporting suspicions of HIV nondisclosure to the authorities, as in instances of suspected child and elder abuse. Subsequently, criminalization adds another restrictive barrier to HIV screening and testing, which negatively impacts patient care and choices, the potential spread of the epidemic, and nursing practice.

Overall, the criminalization of HIV nondisclosure affects the climate of the nursing environment and the kind of information provided in HIV care and counseling. Ultimately, the epidemic thrives as prosecutorial threats can discourage people from knowing and disclosing their status. Nurses must now educate PLWHA and screened patients of the possibility that their confidentiality has limitations, which suggests that nurses should become more engaged in challenging criminalization, as ignoring the harmful consequences of this policy approach not only fails to recognize the advances in medicine that have transformed HIV into a chronic manageable condition, it also ostracizes the rights and dignity of PLWHA. In the next section, we review key criminal cases from the United States, Canada, the United Kingdom, and Australia to illustrate the shifting legal context and to demonstrate the injustices these proceedings inflict upon PLWHA.

REVIEW OF KEY CRIMINAL CASES IN THE UNITED STATES, CANADA, THE UNITED KINGDOM, AND AUSTRALIA

Since 1986 when HIV-specific criminal statutes were first enacted in the United States, an increasing number of countries have applied existing criminal laws and/or created HIV-specific criminal statutes to prosecute PLWHA for nondisclosure (Bernard, 2010; Sullivan & Feldman, 1987). Given our current inadequate ability to systematically track HIV-related prosecutions, it is not possible to determine the actual number of arrests and prosecutions throughout the world. As a result, much of what is known about individual cases comes from media reports. However, it appears that the most active jurisdictions in prosecuting HIV nondisclosure are within high-income countries, including the United States and Canada. As of 2016, the United States and Canada have 345 and 180 documented cases, respectively (AIDS-Free World, 2012; Global Network of People Living with HIV [GNP+] and HIV Justice Network [HIVJN], 2016). The CHLP (2017) has documented 279 U.S. cases between 2008 and 2016 alone. Additionally, both countries have alarming HIV incidence rates for developed nations. In Canada, a new infection occurs every 3 hours, yet 25% of Canadians with HIV are unaware of their diagnosis (Canadian AIDS Treatment Information Exchange [CATIE], 2014). In the United States, there are approximately 50,000 new diagnoses per year and 13% do not know that they are infected (CDC, 2015a).

UNITED STATES OF AMERICA

In the United States, laws vary by state, with some states using HIV-specific laws. Punishments for HIV nondisclosure surpass the sentencing severities of vehicular homicide, driving under the influence (DUI), and reckless endangerment (CHLP, 2013). Additionally, convictions stipulate that PLWHA must be registered as sex offenders, which further complicates their lives and challenges their privacy and employment opportunities (CHLP, 2013). Although the context and content of each case is unique, inconsistencies in legal interpretation and inaccuracies with regard to facts about HIV/AIDS are common.

State of Ohio Appellee v. Roberts

CHLP (2014b) provided the facts of the following case. Roberts appealed his 2003 felonious assault conviction to the Ohio Court of Appeals. The defendant was a 44-year-old African American male who was diagnosed with HIV in 1993. He began HIV treatment and no documentation exists suggesting noncompliance. Although his HIV diagnosis prevented him from joining the Air Force, he graduated with a degree in social work from the University of Akron.

Between September 1999 and April 2000, Roberts began an intimate relationship with TH, a single mother of three. Although they discussed a future together that included marriage, he never disclosed his positive serostatus; the two ended their relationship amicably. Roberts then began a sexual relationship with another single mother, DL, in September 2001. Roberts and DL cohabitated and discussed marriage, but those plans were derailed when DL discovered Roberts' HIV medications. DL and her children moved out of the residence and she filed a complaint with the local authorities, resulting in Roberts' August 2002 indictment. The local paper published news of his arrest, although the article incorrectly described Roberts as homosexual. An anonymous person made TH aware of the article and she filed a similar complaint with the police. Roberts was convicted of one count of felonious assault for nondisclosure of HIV status for his failure to disclose to DL. The charge involving TH was dropped because their relationship ended prior to the enactment of the HIV nondisclosure law. Roberts was sentenced to 4 years of imprisonment, which was upheld on appeal in 2004.

Rhoades v. Iowa State Supreme Court

CHLP (2014a) provided the facts of the following case. Rhoades is a white gay man whose conviction for the criminal transmission of HIV was overturned in 2014. The 34-year-old was diagnosed with HIV in 1998. Although he did not start HIV treatment until 2005, in 2008 he achieved an undetectable viral load. It was at this time that Rhoades met AP, a 22-year-old man, through an online site. Rhoades' online profile indicated that he was HIV negative. Rhoades and AP eventually met and engaged in both oral and anal sex (during which they used a condom). Upon learning that Rhoades was HIV positive (how AP learned this is unreported), AP filed a complaint with the police. Although AP did not contract HIV, counsel advised Rhoades to plead guilty to one count of HIV criminal transmission, for which he received a maximum sentence of 25 years of imprisonment in May 2009. Upon release, he will be on parole for life and will be registered as a sex offender.

Following the trial, Rhoades filed a motion to appeal his sentence, which was suspended and replaced with 5 years of probation in September 2009, by which time he had spent approximately 12 months in prison. On the grounds of ineffective counsel, Rhoades filed a post-conviction relief application in March 2010. The conviction was upheld at the district and appellate judicial levels before landing in the Iowa Supreme Court. At the time, Iowa legislators were revising the state's HIV-specific criminal laws. Arguments were heard in March 2014 and because Rhoades did not demonstrate malicious intent to transmit HIV, as evidenced by condom usage and his undetectable viral load, his conviction was vacated. The case was redirected back to the district courts with instructions to determine a factual basis that would support the original guilty plea; there is no guarantee that Rhoades will not face reindictment.

Campbell v. Texas State Appeals Court

The following case facts were gathered from CHLP (2009). Campbell, a 42-year-old African American homeless man, was found unconscious, smelling of vomit and alcohol by paramedics at 0400. As he roused, he became uncooperative and the medics contacted the Dallas Police Department. Officer Waller arrived at the scene where Campbell remained confrontational. He was arrested for public intoxication and placed in the front passenger seat of the squad car. Upon leaving the scene, Campbell began kicking the dashboard, cursing, and slapping at Waller's hands on the steering wheel. Officer Waller stopped the car, pulled Campbell out, and pepper-sprayed him before calling for assistance. After fellow officers arrived, Waller placed Campbell in the back seat. In the process, Campbell spat at Officer Waller, hitting his eyes and mouth. Officer Waller was not alarmed until Campbell uttered that he had AIDS. Following a blood test, Campbell was found to have HIV, not AIDS.

Campbell testified on his own behalf. He admitted to being diagnosed with HIV at the age of 14. Although he stated his unconsciousness was caused by alcohol and sleeping pills, he denied being confrontational and spitting at Officer Waller. The Clinical Director for the Texas/Oklahoma AIDS Education and Training Center testified that there is a "low risk" of HIV being transmitted through saliva. The expert witness's testimony led to Campbell's 2006 conviction and 35-year sentence for assault with a deadly weapon (HIV). He unsuccessfully appealed his conviction in 2009, again because the courts problematically relied on the expert witness's statement, despite the absence of clinical evidence that HIV can be transmitted through saliva. Campbell remains incarcerated and must serve half of his sentence before being considered for parole.

CANADA

Canada does not have HIV-specific criminal laws and instead uses existing *Criminal Code* legislation to charge individuals for nondisclosure; the most common charge is aggravated sexual assault. The Canadian cases reviewed herein include the three that have gone before the Supreme Court of Canada (SCC) and thus set the country's legal precedent regarding the criminalization of HIV nondisclosure.

R. v. Cuerrier

Cuerrier was diagnosed with HIV in 1992. Shortly thereafter, he began a sexual relationship with KM and then later with BH. KM stated that she explicitly asked Cuerrier about his STI status, but not HIV specifically. The defendant reported that he had tested negative for HIV months earlier. Later in their relationship, they both presented for HIV testing; Cuerrier tested positive, while KM tested negative. They continued their courtship, which included occurrences of unprotected sex for an additional 15 months. Months later, Cuerrier began a new sexual relationship with BH. Although

BH expressed concern over STIs, Cuerrier did not disclose that he was HIV positive. For approximately half of their sexual encounters the couple did not use condoms. BH discovered that Cuerrier was HIV positive and when she confronted him, he admitted so. It is unclear whether or not Cuerrier was compliant with his HIV treatment regimen, but it is of note that neither woman contracted the virus.

Cuerrier was acquitted of two counts of aggravated assault; the judge found that because the women consented to sexual relations with Cuerrier no assault had taken place. While the BC Court of Appeal upheld this verdict, the SCC reversed the decisions of the lower courts and ordered a new trial, citing that because the complainants' consent was gleaned based on fraudulent information, their consent was vitiated. The Supreme Court's decision in *Cuerrier*, commonly referred to as the significant risk test, set the country's legal precedent for all future cases involving HIV nondisclosure for the next 14 years by creating the parameters through which to determine whether or not fraud occurred. First, the accused must have knowledge of their HIV-positive status and of the ways HIV/AIDS can be transmitted. Second, dishonesty must occur, whereby the accused must either deceive the other person about or fail to disclose their HIV-positive status. Third, and most ambiguously defined, is that a "significant risk of serious bodily harm" must arise as a result of the dishonesty. Finally, the accused's dishonesty must be found to have "caused" the person to consent. Ultimately, the Crown must prove that the complainant would not have consented to sexual activity had they been aware of the accused's HIV-positive status.

R. v. Mabior

It is unknown when Mabior, a Sundanese immigrant, was diagnosed with HIV. In 2006, he was charged with aggravated assault after nine women claimed that they were unaware he was HIV-positive before engaging in sexual relations with him. None of the complainants contracted HIV. One of the nine women reported that he denied having an STI when asked. Medical evidence submitted at trial documented that Mabior was compliant with his treatment regimen and that he had a low or undetectable viral load during all of the sexual encounters in question; he did, however, use condoms inconsistently. Eight women testified that they would not have engaged in sexual relations with him if they had known he was HIV-positive.

In 2008, the trial judge ruled that disclosure is necessary even if a condom is used and the viral load is undetectable; Mabior was convicted on six counts of aggravated assault and was sentenced to 14 years of imprisonment. The Manitoba Court of Appeal overturned convictions on four of these counts because either a condom was carefully used or the sex took place when his viral load was undetectable. In 2012, the SCC ruled that significant risk of serious bodily harm as set in the *Cuerrier* decision should be read as "a realistic possibility of transmission of HIV" (p. 18, para. 94). The SCC also determined that the risk of transmission could be reduced so as to justify nondisclosure only when the HIV-positive individual carries a low or undetectable viral load (typically considered 50 copies or less of HIV per cubic ml of blood) *and* a condom is used, thereby setting an even more stringent requirement for disclosure than *Cuerrier*. The SCC found that because the accused had a low viral load at the time of intercourse with three of the complainants, but did not use a condom, the trial judge's convictions on those counts should be maintained. On the fourth count, the SCC ruled to dismiss the appeal because Mabior used a condom and had a low viral load, which they found to negate the realistic possibility of transmission. After completing his sentence, Mabior was deported back to Sudan by the Canadian Border Services Agency.

R. v. DC

DC was compliant with her HIV treatment and her viral load was undetectable. She did not disclose her HIV-positive status to one male partner prior to engaging in their initial sexual encounter. She did, however, disclose her status to him following this first sexual encounter and the couple developed a romantic relationship and remained together for 4 years. When DC ended the relationship in 2004 because the complainant had become violent toward her and her son, upon conviction he retaliated by reporting to police that she had failed to disclose that she was HIV-positive prior to their first sexual encounter. Although DC claimed that they used a condom, the trial judge did not believe her and she was convicted of sexual assault and aggravated assault in 2005. As in *R. v. Mabior*, the Quebec Court of Appeal overruled the conviction on the grounds that nondisclosure of a person's HIV-positive status does not pose a significant risk of transmission when a condom is used or the positive person has an undetectable viral load. The SCC, jointly hearing the *Mabior* and *DC* cases, found that because of the speculative evidence the trial judge used to convict *DC* (i.e., a single hearsay note made 7 years before the trial that no condom was used), the prosecution failed to prove her guilt beyond a reasonable doubt. Accordingly, the verdict was set aside.

UNITED KINGDOM (ENGLAND AND WALES)

The United Kingdom only prosecutes cases where there is actual transmission. Similar to Canada, existing Criminal Code legislation is used and frames nondisclosure as a form of recklessness.

R. v. Dica

Case details were retrieved from www.bailii.org/ew/cases/EWCA/Crim/2004/1103.html

Mohammed Dica was diagnosed with HIV in 1995 and began treatment. Following his diagnosis, Dica had unprotected sexual intercourse with two women, allegedly without disclosing that he was HIV positive. Dica testified that both complainants were aware that he is HIV positive and engaged in consensual sex with him; the complainants later tested positive for HIV. Dica was convicted of two counts of causing grievous bodily harm under s. 20 of the *Offences against the Person Act* (1871) and became the first person to be found guilty of transmitting HIV in England and Wales. He successfully appealed the conviction and the court ordered a new trial.

On appeal, Crown prosecutors argued that Dica acted recklessly as to whether the complainants might be infected. The trial judge determined that whether or not the complainants knew that Dica was HIV positive, their consent was irrelevant and provided no defense. The Court of Appeal ruled that consent to the risk of transmission through consensual sex *is* a valid defense to a charge of reckless transmission, qualifying that consent to the risk of infection would not provide a defense in cases of deliberate infection with intent to cause grievous bodily harm. This decision left unanswered the question of whether or not consenting to unprotected sex equates to consenting to the risk of a STI.

R. v. Konzani

Case details were retrieved from *R. v. Konzani [EWCA] 2005.*

Feston Konzani was born in Malawi in February 1976 and moved to England as an asylum seeker in 1998. In November 2000, he learned that he was HIV positive. On that and subsequent occasions, he was informed of the risks and modes of transmission. He did not disclose his HIV-positive status to the three complainants with whom he had unprotected sexual relations.

The first complainant, DH, met Konzani in 2001 when she was 15 years of age. They had a short-lived sexual relationship, and after taking a blood test in December 2001, DH learned she was HIV positive. The second complainant, RW, met Konzani at church in December 2002 and they began a sexual relationship shortly thereafter. As the relationship deteriorated and eventually ended, RW learned she was pregnant and upon seeking confirmation from a doctor also learned that she was HIV positive. The third complainant, LH, met Konzani in January 2003; he told her that HIV was uncommon in Malawi and did not tell her that he was HIV positive. While they used a condom when they began their sexual relationship, over time Konzani stopped using condoms. When the relationship ended, LH took an HIV test, which came back positive.

Konzani was convicted on three counts of inflicting grievous bodily harm on the three women, contrary to s. 20 of the *Offences Against the Person Act* (1861) and was acquitted of a further such count involving a fourth woman; he was sentenced to a total of 10 years of imprisonment. The question of whether or not consenting to unprotected sex equates to consenting to the risk of infection that went unanswered in *Dica* was later rejected by the Court of Appeal in *R. v. Konzani (2005)*, where a distinction was drawn between "running the risk of transmission" and "willingly" or "consciously" consenting to the risk of transmission of a particular infection, thus establishing that consent must be informed, meaning that the complainant has knowledge of the person's HIV-positive status.

AUSTRALIA

Similar to the United States, criminal legislation relating to HIV transmission and exposure is the responsibility of individual Australian states and territories and the laws vary significantly between the eight different jurisdictions. It is of note that Victoria is the only state with an HIV-specific offense. New South Wales repealed its specific HIV transmission offense (s36 Crimes Act 1900) in 2007, subsuming it within the more general grievous bodily harm section. Like Canada, the states of Victoria and South Australia as well as the Northern Territory extend culpability beyond actual harm to criminalize exposure to HIV.

R. v. Neal

Case details were retrieved from *Neal v. The Queen [2011] VSCA 172* (15 June 2011). www.austlii.edu.au/au/cases/vic/VSCA/2011/172.html

Michael Neal was born on August 26, 1958. He was diagnosed with HIV in June 2000, at which time he was counseled to practice safe sex and to disclose his HIV status to sexual partners. In November 2001, his doctor notified the Department of Human Services (DHS) that he was concerned that Neal was putting others at risk of HIV infection. Between November 2001 and April 2006, the DHS served Neal three letters and four public health orders requiring him to disclose his HIV status and to practice safe sex, which Neal ignored. Neal was originally charged with over 100 offenses, many of which were dropped before the trial, committed against 11 different male complainants. For brevity's sake, we cannot recount the specifics of Neal's sexual encounters with each complainant; it is of note that Neal did not disclose his HIV-positive status, including when directly asked, prior to engaging in unprotected anal sex with each of the 11 complainants. Four of the complainants (ST, NGS, MB, and PW) testified that Neal eventually told them he was HIV positive, that he had organized seroconversion parties, and that told them that he was responsible for infecting many people.

At his committal hearing in March 2007, Neal pleaded guilty to 122 charges and not guilty to 34 charges. In 2008, following a 39-day trial, Neal was convicted of 26 charges. Neal was sentenced to 19 years of imprisonment with parole eligibility after 14 years. Neal won an appeal on the grounds to reconsider technical aspects of the trial judge's directions to the jury, which resulted in a number of his convictions being quashed, including two counts of rape (against two individuals); two counts of administering a drug for the purposes of sexual penetration (associated with the rape charges); and three counts of recklessly endangering a person. His sentence was reduced to 12 years, with eligibility for parole after 9 years.

R. v. Zaburoni

Case details were retrieved from *Zaburoni v. The Queen [2016] HCA 12, 6 April 2016, B69/2015.*

In April 1998, Zaburoni, a Zimbabwean national, was performing as an acrobat with a touring circus in Adelaide. He questioned whether he was HIV positive and sought testing, which revealed a positive result.

The doctor made an appointment for him to attend an infectious disease consultant at the Royal Adelaide Hospital and stressed the importance of using condoms when engaging in sexual intercourse. The doctor noted that he believed Zaburoni understood this advice and that HIV could be transmitted through sexual contact. Zaburoni consulted an infectious diseases physician on three occasions in April and May 1998 and was referred to doctors in Perth, where the circus was next due to perform, so that he could commence antiretroviral therapy. Zaburoni and his then girlfriend attended the Department of Clinical Immunology at the Royal Perth Hospital in July 1998. There they were advised about the natural history of HIV, viral loads, and the need to constantly monitor cell counts. He was referred to the Sexual Health Service for screening for other STIs and for a detailed sexual history to be taken so that his sexual partners could be offered HIV testing. He was prescribed antiretroviral medication and a date was arranged for further review; he did not attend the review, had no further contact with the immunology clinic, and did not undertake antiretroviral therapy.

Zaburoni met the complainant on December 31, 2006. Several weeks later, they commenced a sexual relationship. Before commencing the relationship, the complainant asked if he had been tested for HIV; he told her that he had been tested and was negative. The couple used condoms for approximately 6 weeks, after which they began to have unprotected sexual intercourse. In mid to late 2007, the complainant became ill, exhibiting symptoms of light-headedness, tiredness, colds, vomiting, and diarrhea. She was diagnosed as suffering from glandular fever, although the episode may have been a response to HIV infection known as seroconversion illness. The couple commenced cohabiting shortly thereafter, but their relationship ended in September 2008. In late August 2009, the complainant sought an STI test and telephoned Zaburoni to ask him again if he had HIV, which he denied. On September 1, 2009, the complainant saw Zaburoni, at which time he admitted that he was HIV positive. The complainant's HIV diagnosis was confirmed the next day.

Zaburoni lied to police, stating that when he was diagnosed with HIV in 1998 he was given little information about the condition and had not been told of the need to inform sexual partners of his HIV status. He also said that he took a blood test in April 2005, which returned a negative result. He then admitted that for the test required by the Department of Immigration, he submitted a blood sample taken from his friend. Zaburoni was charged and convicted of transmitting a serious illness with intent to infect, contrary to ss. 317(b) and 317(e) of the *Criminal Code* (1899, Qld), and sentenced to 9 years and 6 months of imprisonment. He appealed the conviction on the grounds that the jury was left to determine intent; by majority ruling, the Queensland Court of Appeal (QCA) dismissed the appeal. In his dissent, Justice Applegarth wrote that while the appellant had a genuine appreciation of the risk of transmission, the evidence did not show whether he knew that risk to be high or low and only supported a finding of recklessness, not intent. The Australia High Court later allowed an appeal against the decision of the QCA on the test for intent and foresight of consequences in the context of HIV transmission. The High Court set aside the orders of the QCA, entered a verdict of guilty on the alternative offense of doing grievous bodily harm (s. 320), and remitted the matter to the Queensland District Court for sentencing.

DISCUSSION AND IMPLICATIONS

These cases demonstrate the variation and inconsistencies in the juridical interpretation of "significant risk" or "realistic possibility" for contracting HIV. With the exception of Campbell, all of the defendants either lied about or failed to disclose that they were HIV positive; however, we contend that this did not present the life-threatening danger that should warrant criminal proceedings, especially when a condom was used or the defendant had a low or undetectable viral load. Campbell's case in particular demonstrates the ignorance and inaccurate information that is too often associated with misunderstandings about HIV risk from differ- ent forms of exposure, namely the negligible risk of transmission for oral sex and sex with a condom. In line with the sentiments of PLWHA and the broader HIV advocacy community, nurses should ally with juridical and grassroots efforts to challenge the criminalization of HIV nondisclo- sure. Together, we must critically ask what is fair and just to punish. This requires considering a number of contextual factors, including whether or not there was an intent to infect; material demonstrations of an ethic of care to protect partners via condom use and/or treatment compliance that secures a low/undetectable viral load; and the sociocultural and relationship contexts within which the PLWHA lives, such as the risk of community ostracizing and the potentiality that the individual might be subject to violence if/when they disclose, rather than solely focusing on (non)disclosure.

Unfortunately, the ongoing moralized HIV/AIDS discourse that is rooted in the fear and stigma born of the moral panic of the early 1980s

(Kilty, 2014) rather than accurate scientific interpretations of the risk of transmission evidenced by current medical evidence is driving policy and judicial decisions. For example, while the Rhoades case demonstrates a more progressive revision of some early judicial outcomes, the Mabior and DC cases set more strict disclosure requirements for PLWHA. Consequently, we suggest that the global repeal of HIV-specific criminal laws and reform to the application of existing criminal code legislation (i.e., must prove malicious intent to infect and transmission must occur) is imperative.

Implications for Judicial Reform

Reform in the context of the criminalization of HIV nondisclosure requires a united campaigning effort from governments, the advocacy and medical communities, and the international public. Perhaps most importantly, it is imperative that laws implicating healthcare are abreast and reflective of current medical practice and science. Lazzarini et al. (2013) suggest that evidence distinguishing between high- and low-risk behaviors, such as those considered in *Mabior, DC,* and *Rhoades*, should spearhead policy changes. We support the position taken by HIV advocates and experts that prosecutions should only occur in cases where there is evidence of the malicious intent to spread HIV *and* where transmission actually occurs (Csete & Elliott, 2011; Jurgens et al., 2009; Latham, 2013; Lazzarini et al., 2013). Prosecutorial guidelines that take up this view have been developed in England, Wales, and Scotland (UNAIDS, 2013) and are currently being developed in Ontario, Canada.

While most criminal cases are framed by prosecutors and media as cases of "deliberate" or "intentional" HIV transmission, the majority have involved neither intent nor transmission (GNP+, 2010). The manner of exposure, viral load, the relationship circumstances of the people involved, and the adoption of safer sex practices like barrier protection are all factors that must be considered to determine intent to transmit. The courts must consider the mind-set of the accused, their understanding of HIV transmission, the risk of harm from disclosure, and if the parties "previously agreed on a level of mutually acceptable risk" (Jurgens et al., 2009, p. 164). Because of the advances in HIV care, all sexual behaviors and exposures do not equate to the same level of risk. In terms of 10,000 exposures, receptive anal intercourse carries the highest risk at 138 while insertive anal intercourse has a risk of 11. Penile-vaginal intercourse has a risk of 8 for receptive and 4 for insertive. Oral intercourse is considered low risk. Biting, spitting, throwing bodily fluids, and sharing sex toys is negligible, meaning that although HIV transmission through these routes is technically possible, it is extremely unlikely and there are no documented cases (Patel et al., 2014; Pretty, Anderson, & Sweet, 1999). Challenging as it may be, policy and/or the repeal of HIV-specific laws should reflect the complex nature of these medical advances. Judicial reform is warranted to preserve public health and promote social justice for PLWHA.

Implications for Public Health

If criminalizing nondisclosure was instituted to end the HIV epidemic, then it has failed miserably. Since 2000, approximately 38.1 million people have become HIV positive, with 2 million new infections occurring in 2014, which UNAIDS (2015) identifies as a 35% reduction from previous years. There is no evidence that this reduction is linked to or supported by criminalization efforts (Gagnon, 2012; Lazzarini et al., 2013; Sweeney et al., 2017) as transmission most often occurs before people are aware of their HIV status (Jurgens et al., 2009). Conduct linked to HIV risk and exposure is complex and socially determined, making behavioral changes due to the threat of prosecutions unrealistic (Gagnon, 2012; Jurgens et al., 2009; Lazzarini et al., 2013). Criminalization works against public health goals in that it fails to reduce HIV exposure behaviors, does not encourage disclosure, and has been found to discourage testing, which may lead PLWHA to refrain from connecting to HIV care practitioners (CHLP, 2013; Jurgens et al., 2009; Lazzarini et al., 2013; Mykhalovskiy, 2011; Sweeney et al., 2017).

The goal of public health is to empower people to practice safer sex, get routine testing to learn their HIV status, and, if positive, comply with treatment and understand the risks associated with different behaviors to try to prevent onward transmission. Public health experts have long advocated that the goal is for everyone to know their HIV status and to perceive every sexual encounter as holding the possibility for infection so that they are encouraged to practice safer sex, but criminalization places the responsibility for the sexual health and safety for both parties solely on the HIV-positive person (Kilty, Orsini, & Balogh, 2017). Flanigan (2014) describes this as non-culpable ignorance, where the plaintiff's responsibility for sexual health and safety is excused. Outside nonconsensual sex and relationships with unequal power relations, as with other STIs, protection against HIV is a mutual decision between two or more parties. Criminalizing HIV nondisclosure does not empower people to "take responsibility for [their] individual sexual health" (CHLP, 2013, p. 1), as "sexual health should be a shared responsibility between sexual partners" (Jurgens et al., 2009, p. 166). While regular discussions between partners regarding sexual health practices and testing may help to foster more open communication about HIV and other STIs, criminalization discourages these discussions.

As aforementioned, medical science in relation to HIV changes rapidly. For example, in July 2012, the Food and Drug Administration (FDA) approved two applications that have major implications for PLWHA. First, rapid testing detects HIV antibodies in 20 minutes for exposures that have occurred within the previous 3 months. Since the testing is conducted using an oral swab, it can be conducted in a clinic or in the privacy of one's own home and was developed for individuals who are unlikely to return to the clinic to receive their results (Francis & Francis, 2013). While there is no guarantee that individuals will take the necessary steps to seek treatment, or get counseling and education if they receive a positive test result, this advancement in testing does create opportunities for people who might fear getting tested in a more public space.

The second FDA approval pertains to prevention. HIV PrEP (pre-exposure prophylaxis) was approved as a daily preventative regimen for HIV-negative persons who engage in high-risk behaviors (CDC, 2014; Francis & Francis, 2013). PrEP is commonly advertised for intravenous drug users (IDUs), men who have sex with men (MSM), people who have multiple sexual partners with inconsistent condom use, those who have sex with serodiscordant partners, and sex workers (CDC, 2014). Extremely costly at $10,000USD per year, PrEP will not be available to all those who may be at risk (Francis & Francis, 2013), but the growing market for PrEP demonstrates that there are individuals who accept a certain degree of HIV risk and exposure—something criminalization denies.

Lastly, criminalization maintains rather than challenges HIV-related stigma and problematically perpetuates much of the erroneous information about the risks of transmission that circulate in the media and in popular discourse. In the era of social media, coverage of criminal prosecutions has allowed and even encouraged sensational and inflammatory commentary and inaccurate information on HIV (e.g., that transmission can occur through biting or spitting) to be widely consumed (CHLP, 2013; Jurgens et al., 2009; Kilty, 2014; Shevory, 2004). In this way, criminalization reinforces ignorance, fear, and myths about HIV, which situates the burden of stigma, rather than science and facts, as a measurement of truth. This leads to and supports the continued social injustice experienced by PLWHA.

CONCLUSION: MOVING TOWARD SOCIAL JUSTICE

The criminalization of HIV nondisclosure creates disadvantages for and promotes discrimination toward PLWHA and may therefore be considered a threat to social justice. Despite the fact that HIV is now considered a chronic manageable condition, criminalization continues to mark it as exceptional in regard to other STIs (Kilty et al., 2017). It is also of note that criminalizing nondisclosure is disproportionately disadvantageous to women who are forced to balance prosecutions with fear of violence (Leham et al., 2014), especially those in heterosexual relationships, where women are more likely to be blamed for contracting the virus (Jurgens et al., 2009). By attempting to force disclosure, even in unsafe situations, criminalization places certain marginalized and at-risk groups—such as women living in unstable environments and/or in potentially violent relationships—at an increased risk of harm and isolation from their families and communities (Jurgens et al., 2009; Leham et al., 2014).

A second marker of criminalization's threat to social justice praxis is the very fact that the application of law and sentencing across cases is inconsistent and unequal. The law is applied broadly and unfairly, which results in punishing blameless behavior such as spitting, biting, and sex with condom use (Jurgens et al., 2009). Racially marginalized and socially and economically disadvantaged HIV-positive persons are disproportionately prosecuted (Gagnon, 2012; Jurgens et al., 2009). Moreover, criminalization constitutes PLWHA as always-already sexual predators who are assumed to be inherently deceitful. People, generally speaking, are not always forthcoming about their sexual practices; adding HIV-related stigma to the picture certainly contributes to legitimately felt fears of violence or retaliation, as seen in the *DC* case. Given that advancements in HIV care and treatment have long been rooted in the activist community and the fact that medical experts and legal and grassroots advocates oppose criminalization, which they contend is an ineffective strategy to promote disclosure and deter onward transmission, we must rethink this political response as an ineffective HIV policy approach (Gagnon, 2012; Kazatchkine, Bernard, & Eba, 2015; UNAIDS, 2013).

It is of note that UNAIDS, the Association of Nurses in AIDS Care (ANAC), and the American Nurses Associations (ANA) agree that the criminalization of HIV nondisclosure violates human rights and jeopardizes public health (Gagnon, 2012). These organizations recognize the injustices and threats that legal actions inflict upon PLWHA, the public, and individual

HIV care and treatment. In an effort to be proactive, Canadian care providers and scientists are uniting to respond to the practice of ill-informed laws and prosecutions. They hope to "assist those in the criminal justice system to understand and interpret medical and scientific evidence regarding HIV" and are working to develop prosecutorial guidelines to better inform prosecutors and defense counsel (Kazatchkine et al., 2015, p. 2). Science has changed our understanding of HIV transmission risk, morbidity, and mortality, but the negative stigma and perception of HIV from the 1980s remains (Kilty, 2014). Each call for judicial reform and repeal hopefully acts as an example that will influence nations, on a global scale, to make similar demands for legal change (ANA, 2016; ANAC, 2015; Gagnon, 2012).

In closing, only time will tell if legislative and judicial officials will begin to recognize the negative impact criminalization has on PLWHA. It is important to note that any dialogue on judicial reform should not be done without consultation with leading medical scientists working in HIV, PLWHA, and their advocates, for the law to accurately consider the realistic nature of the risk of transmission and the harmful, stigmatic consequences of criminalization on the material experiences of PLWHA. These conversations should extend into different cultural communities, homes, families, intimate relationships, and into everyday healthcare encounters; as nurses work on the frontline of HIV care, they must play a leading role in combating HIV-related stigma, shame, and fear.

Repealing HIV-specific laws and carrying out judicial reform that aligns the law with medical science and the development of prosecutorial guidelines will help to combat the stigma associated with HIV. Given that criminalization does nothing to help curb onward transmission and it discourages screening, testing, and disclosure, reform efforts represent the best strategic public health approach to fighting the global epidemic. For one thing is certain, although the epidemic stretches across the globe, it unites the world into a single community fighting for justice for PLWHA.

REFERENCES

AIDS-Free World. (2012). *Criminalization of HIV transmission*. Retrieved from http://www.aidsfreeworld.org/PlanetAIDS/Transmission.aspx

Bernard, E. J. (2010). The evolution of global criminalisation norms: The role of the United States. In E. J. Bernard (Ed.), *HIV and the criminal law*. London, UK: NAM.

Canadian AIDS Treatment Information Exchange. (2014). *Fast facts: HIV/ AIDS in Canada.* Retrieved from http://www.catie.ca/en/pif/spring-2014/ fast-facts-hivaids-canada.html

Center for HIV Law and Policy. (2009). *Campbell v. State, 2009 WL 2025344* (Tex. App. 2009). Retrieved from http://www.hivlawandpolicy.org/resources/ campbell-v-state-2009-wl-2025344-tex-app-2009

Center for HIV Law and Policy. (2013). *Ending and defending against HIV criminalization, a manual for advocates: A legal toolkit: Resources for attorneys handling HIV-related prosecutions.* Retrieved from http://www .aidseducation.org/wp-content/uploads/2014/03/EndingandDefendingAg ainstHIVCriminalization.pdf

Center for HIV Law and Policy. (2014a). *Rhoades v. State of Iowa* (Iowa Supreme Court June 13, 2014). Retrieved from http://www.hivlawandpolicy.org/ resources/rhoades-v-state-iowa-iowa-supreme-court-june-13-2014

Center for HIV Law and Policy. (2014b). *State of Ohio v. Morrondo J. Roberts, 805 N.E.2d 594* (Ohio Ct. App. 2004). Retrieved from http://www .hivlawandpolicy.org/resources/state-ohio-v-morrondo-j-roberts-805 -ne2d-594-ohio-ct-app-2004

Center for HIV Law and Policy. (2015). *Ending and defending against HIV criminalization, a manual for advocates: Vol. 1 State and federal laws and prosecutions* (2nd ed.). Retrieved from http://www.hivlawandpolicy .org/sites/www.hivlawandpolicy.org/files/HIV%20Crim%20Manual% 20%28updated%205.4.15%29.pdf

Center for HIV Law and Policy. (2017). Prosecutions and Arrests for HIV Exposure in the US, 2008–2016. Retrieved from http://www.hivlawandpolicy.org/ resources/arrests-and-prosecutions-hiv-exposure-united-states-2008-2017 -center-hiv-law-policy-2017

Centers for Disease Control and Prevention. (2014). Preexposure prophy-laxis for the prevention of HIV infection in the United States—2014. A clinical practice guideline. Retrieved from http://www.cdc.gov/hiv/pdf/ PrEPguidelines2014.pdf

Centers for Disease Control and Prevention. (2015a). *HIV in the United States: At a glance.* Retrieved from http://www.cdc.gov/hiv/statistics/overview/ ataglance.html

Centers for Disease Control and Prevention. (2015b). *HIV-specific crimi-nal laws.* Retrieved from http://www.cdc.gov/hiv/policies/law/states/ exposure.html

Csete, J., & Elliott, R. (2011). Criminalization of HIV transmission and exposure: In search of rights-based public health alternatives to criminal law. *Future Virology*, 6, 941–950. doi:10.2217/fvl.11.74

Deeks, S. G., Lewin, S. R., & Havlir, D. V. (2013). The end of AIDS: HIV infection as a chronic disease. *Lancet, 382*(9903), 1525–1533. doi:10.1016/S0140-6736(13)61809-7

Flanigan, J. (2014). Non-culpable ignorance and HIV criminalisation. *Journal of Medical Ethics, 40*, 798–801. doi:10.1136/medethics-2012-101119

Francis, J. G., & Francis, L. P. (2013). HIV treatment as prevention: Not an argument for continuing criminalization of HIV transmission. *International Journal of Law in Context, 9*, 520–534. doi:10.107/S1744552313000281

Gagnon, M. (2012). Toward a critical response to HIV criminalization: Remarks on advocacy and social justice. *Journal of Association of Nurses in AIDS Care, 23*, 11–15. doi:10.1016/jana.2011.08.012

Global Network of People Living with HIV. (2010). *The global criminalisation scan report.* Amsterdam, The Netherlands: Author.

Global Network of People Living with HIV and HIV Justice Network. (2016). *Advancing HIV justice 2: Building momentum in global advocacy against HIV criminalisation.* Amsterdam, The Netherlands and London, UK: Author. Retrieved from http://www.hivjustice.net/advancing2

Joint United Nations Programme on HIV/AIDS. (2010). Making the law work for the HIV response: A snapshot of selected laws that support or block universal access to HIV prevention, treatment, care, and support. Retrieved from http://data.unaids.org/pub/BaseDocument/2010/20100728_hr_poster_en.pdf

Joint United Nations Programme on HIV/AIDS. (2013). Ending overly broad criminalisation of HIV non-disclosure, exposure and transmission: Critical scientific, medical and legal considerations. Retrieved from http://www.unaids.org/sites/default/files/media_asset/20130530_Guidance_Ending_Criminalisation_0.pdf

Joint United Nations Programme on HIV/AIDS. (2015). *Fact sheet: 2015 global statistics.* Retrieved from http://www.unaids.org/sites/default/files/media_asset/20150901_FactSheet_2015_en.pdf

Jurgens, R., Cohen, J., Cameron, E., Burris, S., Clayton, M., Elliott, R., ... Cupido, D. (2009). Ten reasons to oppose the criminalization of HIV exposure or transmission. *Reproductive Health Matters, 17*, 163–172. doi:10.1016/S0968-8080(09)34462-6

Kazatchkine, C., Bernard, E., & Eba, P. (2015). Ending overly broad HIV criminalization: Canadian scientists and clinicians stand for justice. *Journal of the International AIDS Society, 18,* 1–2. doi:10.7448/IAS.18.1.20126

Kilty, J. M. (2014). Dangerous liaisons, a tale of two cases: Constructing women accused of HIV nondisclosure as threats to the (inter)national body politic. In J. M. Kilty (Ed.), *Within the confines: Women and the law in Canada* (pp. 271–292). Toronto, ON, Canada: Women's Press.

Kilty, J. M., Orsini, M., & Balogh, P. (2017). Critical bioethics in the time of epidemic: The case of the criminalization of HIV/AIDS nondisclosure in Canada. *Aporia, 9*(1), 9–18.

Latham, S. R. (2013). Time to decriminalize HIV status. *Hastings Center Report, 5,* 12–13. doi:10.1002/hast.205

Lazzarini, Z., Galletly, C. L., Mykhalovskiy, E., Harsono, D., O'Keefe, E., Singer, M., . . . Levine, R. J. (2013). Criminalization of HIV transmission and exposure: Research and policy agenda. *American Journal of Public Health, 103,* 1350–1353. doi:10.2105/AJPH.2013.301267

Lehman, J. S., Carr, M. H., Nichol, A. J., Ruisanchez, A., Knight, D. W., Langford, A. E., . . . Mermin, J. H. (2014). Prevalence and public health implications of state laws that criminalize potential HIV exposure in the United States. *AIDS Behavior, 18,* 997–1006. doi:10.1007/s10461-014-0724-0

Mykhalovskiy, E. (2011). The problem of "significant risk": Exploring the public health impact of criminalizing HIV non-disclosure. *Social Science and Medicine, 73,* 668–675. doi:10.1016/j.socscimed.2011.06.051

O'Bryne, P. (2011). HIV, nursing practice, and the law: What does HIV criminalization mean for practicing nurses? *Journal of the Association of Nurses in AIDS Care, 22,* 339–344. doi:10.1061/j.ana.2011.02.002

Patel, P., Borkowf, C. B., Brooks, J. T., Lasry, A., Lansky, A., & Mermin, J. (2014) Estimating per-act HIV transmission risk: A systematic review. *AIDS, 28*(10), 1509–1519. doi:10.1097/QAD.0000000000000298

Pretty, L. A., Anderson, G. S., & Sweet, D. J. (1999). Human bites and the risk of human immunodeficiency virus transmission. *American Journal of Forensic Medicine and Pathology, 20*(3), 232–239.

Sanders, C. (2014). Discussing the limits of confidentiality: The impact of criminalizing HIV nondisclosure on public health nurses' counseling practices. *Public Health Ethics, 7,* 253–260. doi:10.1093/phe/phu032

Shevory, T. (2004). *Notorious H.I.V.: The media spectacle of Nushawn Williams.* Minneapolis: University of Minnesota Press.

Sullivan, S. K., & Feldman, M. C. (1987). Imposing criminal liability on those who knowingly transmit the AIDS virus: A recommendation for legislative action. *University of Dayton Law Review, 13*(3), 489–509.

Sweeney, P., Gray, S. C., Purcell, D. W., Sewell, J., Surendera Babu, A., Tarver, B. A.,… Mermen, J. (2017). Association of HIV diagnosis rates and laws criminalizing HIV exposure in the United States. *AIDS, 31*(10), 1483–1488. doi:10.1097/QAD.0000000000001501

LEGAL CASES

Neal v. The Queen [2011] VSCA 172.

R. v. Cuerrier, [1998] 2 SCR 371; [1996] BCJ No 2229 (QL), 83 BCAC 295; (1995), 26 WCB (2d) 378.

R. v. Konzani [EWCA] 2005.

R. v. Mabior, 2012 SCC 47; [2010] MJ No 308, 2010 MBCA 93; [2008] MBQB 201, 230 Man R (2d) 184.

Zaburoni v. The Queen [2016] HCA 12, 6 April 2016, B69/2015.

Global Health Policy Considerations: Autism Spectrum Disorder

M'Lyn Spinks

Autism spectrum disorders (ASD) are defined by the *Diagnostic and Statistical Manual of Mental Disorders* (DSM) as a diverse set of neurodevelopmental disorders characterized by various persistent patterns of behaviors in childhood (American Psychiatric Association [APA], 2013). These behaviors include deficiencies in verbal and nonverbal communication, socio-emotional reciprocity, and restricted patterns of behavior, which are usually repetitive, and sometimes violent (APA, 2013; Ziats & Rennert, 2016). With an estimated, albeit highly debated, worldwide prevalence rate of 1% to 2% of children and, for many, a life-long prognosis of dependence, ASD is a global healthcare concern that calls for worldwide collaboration in health policy (Centers for Disease Control and Prevention, 2016; Özerk, 2016; Steinhausen, Jensen, & Lauritsen, 2016). Worldwide collaboration among providers, parents, and people with autism can lead to advances in early identification, effective interventions, and potential resolutions to address the complex needs of this population and their caregivers within the multicultural setting of current society. This chapter provides current ASD diagnostic information, prevalence, and factors affecting treatment options in the United States and abroad. It also discusses the relationship between health policy and healthcare systems that create barriers in access to care from a global perspective. While the actual barriers in each country discussed may have different characteristics, the factors supporting or eliminating them have constituent components. Only through a discussion of these relationships, barriers, and their associated factors can there be sustained improvement in the health outcomes and quality of life for clients on the autism spectrum and their caregivers.

DESCRIPTION AND PREVALANCE OF AUTISM

Worldwide identification of children with ASD has resulted in efforts by countries at all economic levels to integrate health policy legislation to improve access to ASD assessment, diagnosis, and treatment (Australian Bureau of Statistics, 2014; Elsabbagh et al., 2012). These efforts are motivated by the desire of community leaders and individuals to identify and implement strategies that will improve outcomes, positively impact the quality of life, and reduce care burden for families and communities affected by the diagnosis of autism. Much like obtaining a diagnosis of ASD, an often arduous and complicated endeavor, estimating the global presence of ASD is an extremely complex and challenging process yet vital to the success of healthcare and its related health policies. Inconsistencies in concept descriptions plagued early epidemiological studies and inhibited the reporting of accurate ASD prevalence rates (Lotter, 1966; Wing, Yeates, Brierly, & Gould, 1976). These inconsistencies in defining and describing ASD led to lower estimations due to an absence of the milder ASD phenotypes and children with a normative intelligence quotient (IQ; Elsabbagh et al., 2012; Wing & Gould, 1979). Thus a discussion of health policy impacted by ASD prevalence must begin with an accurate conceptualization of autism.

DESCRIPTION

Since the time of the first descriptions of autism by Kanner (1943) and after many modifications in the diagnostic description of autism, a current definition of autism has been formalized by the APA. The current definition of autism contains two essential clinical features: sustained "social and communication defects" and "fixed interests and repetitive behaviors" occurring on a continuum from mild to severe (APA, 2013, p. xlii). This concept of a continuum from mild to severe is the key component to an understanding of ASD yet complicates identification and accurate clinical diagnosis. A combination of attributes within each of these domains, as determined by a validated, standardized measure, accompanied by an observational assessment by a highly trained provider, determines an accurate clinical diagnosis of ASD (Dr. H. Ormand, personal communication, Feburary 27, 2017). In the social and communication domain, the patient must demonstrate difficulty or an inability to perform certain actions irrespective of a general developmental delay. In the fixed interest and repetitive behaviors domain, the patient must demonstrate two of the associated characteristics. These include: (a) stereotypical or repetitive speech, movement, or use of objects; (b) ritualistic patterns of verbal or nonverbal behaviors with resistance to change; (c) abnormally intense focus on extremely restricted interests; or (d) "hypo- or hyper-reactivity to sensory input or unusual interest in sensory aspects of the environment" (Ziats & Rennert, 2016, p. 2). Now with a clear understanding of ASD, we can address the issue of prevalence.

PREVALENCE

Prevalence estimates for ASD worldwide are approximately 1% to 2% of all children (Elsabbagh et al., 2012). The value of accurate prevalence data is its contribution to the advancement of relevant research foci and the strategic development of policy-influencing services. Yet efforts to obtain accurate prevalence rates are, at times, siloed in cultural values of the West and within high-income, high-resource countries (Murillo, Shih, Rosanoff, Daniels, & Reagon, 2016; Samms-Vaughan, 2014). Despite development of a detailed description of the diagnosis, multiple studies have found that screening tool selection, severity of symptoms, socioeconomic status, and culture influence the perception of these attributes, thus impacting prevalence data (Ravindran & Myers, 2012).

SCREENING TOOL SELECTION

Elsabbagh et al. (2012) conducted a systematic review of epidemiological prevalence surveys including both ASD and pervasive developmental disorders (PDD) in order to more accurately capture cases across the spectrum of autism. The review identifies the utilization of up to

11 different screening tools in the selected prevalence surveys (Elsabbagh et al., 2012). Elsabbagh et al. recorded a disparity within these recorded prevalence rates ranging from as great as 186.7/10,000 to as little as 27.6/10,000.

SEVERITY OF SYMPTOMS

The severity of symptoms influences prevalence rates due to the subtlety of diagnostic symptoms and provider perspectives of the screening process (Emerson, Morrel, & Neece, 2016; Johnson, 2016). Ward, Sullivan, and Gilmore (2016) found that 50% of primary care providers in the United States do not perform a routine screening for ASD. Pediatricians, while more likely to incorporate developmental screening practices than other providers, state "lack of time, familiarity, training, confidence, and knowledge of available resources" as barriers to routine screening (Self, Parham, & Rajagopalan, 2015). Despite improvements in screening practices over the past decade, the data continue to highlight issues with accurate prevalence rates due to inconsistent screening practices, difficulties in diagnosis, initiation of treatment, and engagement with specialists that often serve as the access point for researchers to obtain their participants.

Country's Socioeconomic Status

The majority of ASD research originates in high-income countries such as the United States and UK (Stewart & Lee, 2017). For research to accurately reflect the global prevalence of autism, and thus correctly influence international policy, elimination of information gaps in low- to middle-income countries (LMIC) is a necessity. The unique factors in LMIC countries include an overall lack of healthcare, deficits in ASD awareness among both providers and laypersons, and absence of economic feasibility of specialty healthcare systems (Stewart & Lee, 2017). Complicated assessment tools and insufficient numbers of specialists to execute them with high specificity compound the existing financial limitations in these countries. This lack of tools and providers to use them increases reliance on parent/caregiver report to ascertain developmental concerns and consequently yields limitations in reliability of a diagnosis.

CULTURE

Bronfenbrenner's (1994) ecological model provides a rationale for prioritizing the influence of culture on assessments of development. Based on propositions of the ecological model, accurate prevalence rates would require a culturally sensitive perspective. An example of this requirement is seen in Soto et al.'s (2015) systematic review isolating international ASD studies from Central and South America, Europe, Asia, Southeast Asia, and the Middle East. Soto et al. noted that studies using adapted screening tools rarely explicate the process of cultural tool adaptation, infrequently adhere to recommended guidelines for use, and often yield inconsistent psychometric properties between original tools and their adapted versions. Culturally adapted tools, according to Soto et al., would help tool administrators to avoid either overreporting or underreporting cases—factors which prohibit successful policy strategies necessary for an effective and appropriate systemic response.

Additional cultural factors that influence prevalence rates center around perceptions of illness and research, stigma, and the ability to identify cases. Viewing ASD as a parenting capability issue often leads to familial isolation as the child is shielded from the public, friends, and even family. This social isolation, potentiated by actual and perceived experiences of stigmatism, is associated with feelings of shame and guilt (Burkett, Morris, Anthony, Shambley-Ebron, & Manning-Courtney, 2016; Dababnah & Parish, 2013). Incorrectly identifying the symptoms of ASD as a deficiency on the part of the parent or caregiver, common in both Western and Eastern cultures, results in lower published prevalence rates and fewer identified cases (Kang-Yi, Grinker, & Mandell, 2013; Sousa, 2011).

Daley, Singhal, and Krishnamurthy (2013) identified cultural factors specific to India. Deeply held philosophies of offspring, particularly in Eastern cultures, impact the availability of census data. In India, female infanticide alters gender-specific birth rates, while abortion of disabled infants contributes to a disproportionate number of unaffected infants, thus creating skewed data (Daley et al., 2013; Girimaji & Kommu, 2016). Other cultural factors that influence prevalence rate records include fear of being denied educational support and rejection as a suitable marriage partner (Daley et al., 2013; Eseigbe et al., 2015). Disability has the power to affect all aspects of life in any culture. For some cultures, disability is more of an inconvenience with minor societal influence. In other cultures, however, it can result in parental denial, failure to report, or even the inability to request assistance due to fears of societal rejection, isolation, and ridicule. These disparate views of disability affect more than just prevalence. The value and importance of a person, with or without a disability, plays an integral part in policy making.

DISABILITY POLICIES AND AUTISM SPECTRUM DISORDERS

Overwhelming research supporting the global prevalence of autism motivates some countries to implement policies that recognize ASD as a disability, increase awareness for allocation of resources for the care of people on the spectrum, and provide a legal framework for the protection of the rights of individuals with ASD. In the United States, policies within the Individuals with Disabilities Education Improvement Act (IDEA) provide for early intervention services and equal educational opportunities where available (U.S. Government Printing Office, 2004). Countries besides those in North America and Europe and Australia have policies that recognize the rights of the disabled as well. Though many other countries have similar policies, delays in implementation may be due to their philosophies of personhood, redistribution and allocation of resources, and the role of the individual in the community rather than as a statement of disagreement with disability policy (Stein, 2011). China, for example, known for its collectivist culture, supported international United Nations (UN) policies for the protection of disability rights long before its implementation of the Disability Discrimination Ordinance (DDO) in 1996 that provides for equal opportunities in education (Equal Opportunities Commission, 2011; Stein, 2011).

In India, as in China, similar barriers to access to care exist. Constituting one of the largest Southeast Asian countries, India has many regulatory and legislative similarities with China (Minhas et al., 2015). India recognized the rights of the disabled in the mid-1990s with the Equal Opportunities, Protection of Rights and Full Participation Act (Ministry of Law, Justice and Company Affairs; Legislative Branch, 1996). Following this policy in 1999 was the inclusion of autism as a unique developmental disorder (Ministry of Law, Justice and Company Affairs; Legislative Branch, 1999). Despite meaningful legislation that identifies and offers support to children with ASD, Minhas et al. (2015) explain that in India only the most populated urban areas have health services and even fewer services for identification or treatment for autism.

Iranian policy makers and citizens also experience this conundrum. According to Shooshtari et al. (2014), there is a disconnect between research, policy, and practice among stakeholders of developmental disabilities issues. While legislators, providers, and citizens are in agreement with supporting the creation and presence of supportive legislation for physical health, developmental, intellectual, and behavioral needs are often neglected. This physical health focus has led to major improvements in access to services, infant mortality, and life expectancy (Sharifi et al., 2016). Policies involving disability, however, lag behind and do not provide the resources for implementation of services in developmental disabilities (Sharifi et al., 2016). Due to a lack of supportive policy and funding, the Iranian State Welfare Organization offers day care in large urban locations for those children who are unable to attend school due to the severity of their disability; unfortunately, the cost is prohibitive for all but the most affluent (Samadi & McConkey, 2011). Due to the financial burden and social stigma of ASD, parents often elect private tutoring and traditional healers versus professional providers and services (Sharifi et al., 2016). As these children enter adulthood, without a national mental health policy, there are no more facilities to provide care, housing, or employment (Sharifi et al., 2016).

As evident in the actions of the UN and its members, there is a global desire to respect, support, and promote the health and well-being of all persons with disabilities. Yet policies and legislative support for an early identification process or the provision of access to treatment for children with ASD are only applicable if the resources to implement these strategies are available (Hue, 2012; Song, Giannotti, & Reichow, 2013). A review of financial factors provides additional insight into the interrelationship between these components.

FINANCIAL POLICIES AND ASD

Many evidence-based options exist in the treatment of ASD. An interdisciplinary search of multiple databases limited to between 2012 and 2017 located 651 peer-reviewed journal articles containing or referencing ASD interventions, treatments, or therapies. These articles included behavioral, educational, and psychological interventions focusing on the primary parental and societal concerns of socialization, communication, education, and health outcomes. While reviewing and comparing these interventions is beyond the scope of this paper, awareness of the disparity in treatment approaches is helpful in understanding the amount of information required to create, implement, and evaluate health policy. Intricately involved in a discussion of interventions is the necessary component of cost. While the psychology, education, medicine, and ancillary health communities from predominantly Western countries look for interventions, the global political community is attempting to understand its role and place in the primary issues involved in the care of people affected by autism.

GLOBAL FINANCIAL POLICIES

As with prevalence rates, the determination of a country's resource capabilities and its designation within political, economic, and healthcare performance analyses affects both national and international finance policies. It is within these analyses of fiscal capabilities that resource support needs can be accessed and obtained. The World Health Organization (WHO) ranks countries by the performance outcomes of their health-care system. These outcome measures of healthcare performance are the foundation from which the WHO facilitates equitable economic, social, and environmental development (WHO, 2016, p. v). The UN Department of Economic and Social Affairs determines country rank using basic economic conditions (Economic Groupings, 2016). These UN rankings provide vital data to researchers, analysts, and government agencies for statistical analysis and research while remaining disconnected to any legal status or opinion by the UN (United Nations Conference on Trade and Development [UNCTD], 2016). Lastly, country rankings determined by the World Bank (WB) are generated based on gross individual income (World Bank, 2017). Calculations based on the WB figures help the bank's leaders prioritize and attain the goals necessary to achieve the purposes and goals of the WB. The goals of the WB consist of a reduction in global poverty and supportive measures to increase the income growth of people living in poverty in every country on the planet (World Bank, 2014). Based on one or more of these rankings, low- and middle-resource countries have greater access to financial support for research, system development, implementation, and future evaluation of issues of healthcare. Clarification of the global connection between finance and healthcare now facilitates appreciation of the narrower perspective of finances and ASD.

IMPACT OF FINANCIAL FACTORS ON ASD TREATMENT

Research indicates that reducing age at diagnosis and removing delays in treatment significantly improves outcomes and reduces the lifelong caregiving burden to countries and individuals responsible for the care of this population (Horlin, Falkmer, Parsons, Albrecht, & Falkmer, 2014; Webb, Jones, Kelly, & Dawson, 2014). David Mandell, ScD, of the University of Pennsylvania, and Martin Knapp, PhD, of the London School of Economics, presented their findings in 2012 on the economic impact of ASD on the United States. Their research summarized an estimated annual cost of ASD to the nation of $137 billion per year, an amount that exceeds the gross domestic product of over 139 countries (Autism Speaks, 2012). A valuable asset in countries like the United States is a nationally funded organization such as the Centers for Medicare and Medicaid Services (CMS). Depending on the level of assistance dictated by individual state legislation, the CMS can provide financial support to compensate for, at minimum, a portion of ASD healthcare costs (Hall-Lande, Hewitt, & Moseley, 2011; Leslie et al., 2017; Miller, Merryman, Eskow, & Chasson, 2016).

Similar in structure and function, the Australian welfare system contains policies to address care and needs of the person with a disability (McClure, Sinclair, & Aird, 2015). Leigh and Du (2015) offer documentation of projected comparative costs in Australia. Based on annual medical, nonmedical, and productivity costs, they estimate the projected national expenditure for ASD in 2025 will reach close to $500 billion (Leigh & Du, 2015). Additional research into adult ASD health outcomes supports the financial benefits of early intervention, thus providing increased motivation for health policy to include early identification and immediate access to care (Barbaro & Halder, 2016; Penner et al., 2015). Understanding the impact that policy can have on facilitating and financing early diagnosis and access to intervention is therefore critical. International and national policy can provide a framework within which to identify and provide cost reduction strategies while also including an evaluative process for further revision as healthcare needs and costs change.

EARLY DIAGNOSIS

Numerous research studies substantiate the mandate by the American Academy of Pediatrics (AAP) for universal screening and subsequent early intervention (Spjut Jansson et al., 2016; Webb et al., 2014). Conversely, the U.S. Preventive Services Task Force (Siu, 2016) and the National Health Service of the United Kingdom (United Kingdom National Screening Committee, 2012) denounced universal screening, which may potentially harm children, without some degree of parental or clinical concern.

However, countries such as India, categorized as a lower-middle income country by the World Bank (2017) and as a developing country by both the WHO and the UN, are in a precarious position when deciding which policy is applicable to their country. Despite a conservative estimate of 2 million children in India with autism, there is still no comprehensive public awareness of autism (Mhatre, Bapat, & Udani, 2015). Providers, policy makers, and other stakeholders in Indian health are aware of the recommendations for ASD care, yet they are still in the process of organizing and prioritizing limited healthcare resources (World Bank, 2017). Nair et al. (2010) identified that primary concerns for pediatric healthcare in India remained centered around prenatal and perinatal care, immunization support, and basic nutritional needs.

ACCESS TO INTERVENTION

Nova Scotia, ranked 9th for quality of life by the UN, 30th in healthcare efficiency by the WHO, and classified as a high-income economy, would seem to have everything it needs (Tandon, Murray, Lauer, & Evans, 2000; World Bank, 2017; UNCTD, 2016). And yet, with all of these accolades, Nova Scotia has many of the same issues in ASD access to care related to age at diagnosis and intervention as both high- and low-resource countries (Frenette et al., 2011; Thomas, Parish, Rose, & Kilany, 2012). Because ASD involves a spectrum of symptoms ranging from mild to severe, a delayed diagnosis subsequently leads to a delay in treatment (Zwaigenbaum et al., 2015). According to Dr. H. Ormand of the Kennedy Krieger Institute, these delays create significant barriers to an optimum developmental trajectory, hinder future adaptation by children with ASD, and often result in prolonged treatment protocols, extensive caregiver burden, and reduced adaptation as an adult (Dr. H. Ormand, personal communication, February 27, 2017).

CONCLUSION

A compelling feature of current global ASD healthcare policies is their presence and efficacy. Policies are created to "solve intractable problems" (Milstead, 2013). The problems and issues surrounding ASD have been recognized and discussed here. Policies have been found among most countries to address these problems. However, the success or failure of these policies can only be determined through an evaluative process that incorporates the goals and objectives of these policies. An effective evaluative process for policy provides results of systematic and validated research into patient outcomes, satisfaction scores bestowed by stakeholders, and reduction in the fiscal burden of the disorder for both individuals and countries. Despite the standardized evaluation methods created by organizations such as the WHO and the UN, it remains difficult to determine an accurate global understanding of the presence and impact of policy. This difficulty lies in the fact that an overwhelming majority of legislative and regulatory documentation originates in high-income countries with well-established integration between systems of policy and healthcare. Yet without a standardized method of prevalence determination, lack of uniformity in provider training, and varying levels of public knowledge about ASD, these policies may be misunderstood, poorly funded, and underutilized in other settings. All of these issues coalesce into a call for a comprehensive system of collaboration between researchers, providers, and caregivers. By joining forces at both the national and international levels, stakeholders can improve efforts to identify, classify, organize, and evaluate health policies and their efficacy in improving healthcare for the person with ASD.

REFERENCES

American Psychiatric Association. (2013). *Diagnostic and statistical manual of mental disorders* (5th ed.). Arlington, VA: American Psychiatric Publishing.

Australian Bureau of Statistics. (2014, June 3). *4428.0—Autism in Australia, 2012*. Retrieved from http://www.abs.gov.au/ausstats/abs@.nsf/Latestproducts/4428.0Main%20Features32012?opendocument&tabname=Summary&prodno=4428.0&issue=2012&num=&view=

Autism Speaks. (2012, July 24). *Autism's costs to the nation reach $137 billion a year*. Retrieved from https://www.autismspeaks.org/site-wide/economic-costs

Barbaro, J., & Halder, S. (2016). Early identification of autism spectrum disorder: Current challenges and future global directions. *Current Developmental Disorders Reports, 3*(1), 67–74. doi:10.1007/s40474-016-0078-6

Bronfenbrenner, U. (1994). Ecological models of human development. In T. Husen, & T. N. Postlethwaite (Eds.), *The International Encyclopedia of Education*. Oxford, UK: Pergamon.

Burkett, K., Morris, E., Anthony, J., Shambley-Ebron, D., & Manning-Courtney, P. (2016). Parenting African American children with autism: The influence of respect and faith in mother, father, single-, and two-parent care. *Journal of Transcultural Nursing: Official Journal of the Transcultural Nursing Society.* doi:10.1177/1043659616662316

Centers for Disease Control and Prevention. (2016, July 11). *Autism spectrum disorders*. Retrieved from https://www.cdc.gov/ncbddd/autism/data.html

Communication from the Commission to the European Parliament, the Council, the European Economic and Social Committee, and the Committee of the Regions. (2010). *European Disability Strategy 2010–2020: A renewed commitment to a barrier-free Europe*. Retrieved from http://eur-lex.europa.eu/LexUriServ/LexUriServ.do?uri=COM:2010:0636:FIN:en:PDF

Daley, T. C., Singhal, N., & Krishnamurthy, V. (2013). Ethical considerations in conducting research in autism spectrum disorders in low and middle income countries. *Journal of Autism and Developmental Disorders, 43*, 2002–2014. doi:10.1007/s10803-012-1750-2

Elsabbagh, M., Divan, G., Koh, Y.-J., Kim, Y. S., Kauchali, S., Marcín, C., ... Fombonne, E. (2012). Global prevalence of autism and other pervasive developmental disorders. *Autism Research, 5*, 160–179. doi:10.1002/aur.239

Emerson, N., Morrell, H., & Neece, C. (2016). Predictors of age of diagnosis for children with autism spectrum disorder: The role of a consistent source of medical care, race, and condition severity. *Journal of Autism and Developmental Disorders, 46*(1), 127–138. doi:10.1007/s10803-015-2555-x

Equal Opportunities Commission. (2011). *Disability discrimination ordinance: Code of practice on education*. Retrieved from https://www.gov.hk/en/about/abouthk/factsheets/docs/eoc.pdf

Eseigbe, E. E., Nuhu, F. T, Sheikh, T. L., Eseigbe, P., Sanni, K. A., & Olisah, V. O. (2015). Knowledge of childhood autism and challenges of management among medical doctors in Kaduna state, Northwest Nigeria. *Autism Research and Treatment, 2015*, 1–6. doi:10.1155/2015/892301

Frenette, P., Dodds, L., MacPherson, K., Flowerdew, G., Hennen, B., & Bryson, S. (2013). Factors affecting the age at diagnosis of autism spectrum disorders in Nova Scotia, Canada. *Autism, 17*(2), 184–195. doi:10.1177/1362361311413399

Girimaji, S. C., & Kommu, J. V. S. (2016). Intellectual disability in India: Recent trends in care and services. *Health Care for People with Intellectual and Developmental Disabilities Across the Lifespan*, 461–470. doi:10.1007/978-3-319-18096-0_39

Hall-Lande, J., Hewitt, A., & Mosely, C. (2011). A national review of home and community based services (HCBS) for individuals with autism spectrum disorders. *Policy Research Brief, 21*(3), 1–11. Retrieved from https://ici.umn .edu/products/prb/213/213.pdf

Horlin, C., Falkmer, M., Parsons, R., Albrecht, M. A., & Falkmer, T. (2014). The cost of autism spectrum disorders. *PLoS One, 9*(9), e106552. doi:10.1371/ journal.pone.0106552

Hue, M. (2012). Inclusion practices with special educational needs students in a Hong Kong secondary school: Teachers' narratives from a school guidance perspective. *British Journal of Guidance and Counselling, 40*(2), 143–156. doi:10.1080/03069885.2011.646950

Johnson, N. L. (2016). Translating research to practice for children with autism spectrum disorder: Part I: Definition, associated behaviors, prevalence, diagnostic process, and interventions. *Journal of Pediatric Health Care, 30*(1), 15–26. doi:10.1016/j.pedhc.2015.09.008

Kang-Yi, C., Grinker, R., & Mandell, D. (2013). Korean culture and autism spectrum disorders. *Journal of Autism and Developmental Disorders, 43*(3), 503. doi:10.1007/s10803-012-1570-4

Kanner, L. (1943). Autistic disturbances of affective contact. *Nervous Child, 2*, 217–250.

Lotter, V. (1966). Epidemiology of autistic conditions in young children: I. Prevalence. *Social Psychiatry, 1*, 124–137. doi:10.1007/BF00584048

Leigh, J. P., & Du, J. (2015). Brief report: Forecasting the economic burden of autism in 2015 and 2025 in the United States. *Journal of Autism and Developmental Disorders, 45*(12), 4135–4139. doi:10.1007/s10803-015-2521-7

Leslie, D., Iskandarani, K., Velott, D., Agbese, E., Stein, B., Dick, A., & Mandell, D. (2017). Medicaid waivers targeting children with autism spectrum disorder reduce the need for parents to stop working. *Health Affairs, 36*(2), 282–288. doi:10.1377/hlthaff.2016.1136

McClure, P., Sinclair, S., & Aird, W. (2015, February 25). *A new system for better employment and social outcomes.* Australian Government, Department of Social Services. Retrieved from https://www.dss.gov.au/review-of-australias-welfare-system

Mhatre, D., Bapat, D., & Udani, V. (2015). Long-term outcomes in children diagnosed with autism spectrum disorders in India. *Journal of Autism and Developmental Disorders, 46*(3), 760–772. doi:10.1007/s10803-015-2613-4

Miller, N., Merryman, M. B., Eskow, K. G., & Chasson, G. S. (2016). State design and use of Medicaid 1915(c) waivers and related benefits to provide services to children and youth with autism spectrum disorder. *American Journal on Intellectual and Developmental Disabilities, 121*(4), 295–311. doi:10.1352/1944-7558-121.4.295

Milstead, J. (2013). *Health policy and politics: A nurse's guide* (5th ed.). Burlington, MA: Jones and Bartlett.

Minhas, A., Vajaratkar, V., Divan, G., Hamdani, S. U., Leadbitter, K., Taylor, C., … Rahman, A. (2015). Parents' perspectives on care of children with autistic spectrum disorder in South Asia—Views from Pakistan and India. *International Review of Psychiatry, 27*(3), 247–256. doi:10.3109/09540261.2015.1049128

Ministry of Law, Justice and Company Affairs; Legislative Branch. (1996). *Equal Opportunities, Protection of Rights and Full Participation Act 1995* (Report No.1). New Delhi, India: Author.

Ministry of Law, Justice and Company Affairs; Legislative Branch. (1999). *The National Trust for the Welfare of Persons with Autism, Cerebral Palsy, Mental Retardation and Multiple Disabilities Act, 1999* (Report No. 44). New Delhi, India: Author.

Murillo, L., Shih, A., Rosanoff, M., Daniels, A. M., & Reagon, K. (2016). The role of multi-stakeholder collaboration and community consensus building in improving identification and early diagnosis of autism in low-resource settings. *Australian Psychologist, 51*(4), 280–286. doi:10.1111/ap.12226

Nair, M. K. C., Princly, P., Leena, M. L., Swapna, S., Kumari I. L., Preethi, R., … Russell, P. S. S. (2014). CDC Kerala 17: Early detection of developmental delay/disability among children below 3 y in Kerala—A cross sectional survey. *Indian Journal of Pediatrics, 81*(2), 156–160. doi:10.1007/s12098-014-1579-0

Özerk, K. K. (2016). The issue of prevalence of autism/ASD. *International Electronic Journal of Elementary Education, 9*(2), 263–305.

Penner, M., Rayar, M., Bashir, N., Roberts, S. W., Hancock-Howard, R. L., & Coyte, P. C. (2015). Cost-effectiveness analysis comparing pre-diagnosis autism spectrum disorder (ASD)–targeted intervention with Ontario's Autism Intervention Program. *Journal of Autism and Developmental Disorders, 45*(9), 2833–2847. doi:10.1007/s10803-015-2447-0

Ravindran, N., & Myers, B. J. (2012). Cultural influences on perceptions of health, illness, and disability: A review and focus on autism. *Journal of Child and Family Studies,* (2), 311–319. doi:10.1007/s10826-011-9477-9

Samms-Vaughan, M. E. (2014). The status of early identification and early intervention in autism spectrum disorders in lower- and middle-income countries. *International Journal of Speech-Language Pathology, 16*(1), 30–35. doi:10.3109/17549507.2013.866271

Samadi, S. A. & McConkey, R. (2011). Autism in developing countries: Lessons from Iran. *Autism Research and Treatment, 2011,* 1–11. doi:10.1155/2011/145359

Self, T., Parham, D., & Rajagopalan, J. (2015). Autism spectrum disorder early screening practices: A survey of physicians. *Communication Disorders Quarterly, 36*(4), 195–207. doi:10.1177/1525740114560060

Sharifi, V., Mojtabai, R., Shahnvar, Z., Alaghband-Rad, J., Zarafshan, H., & Wissow, L. (2016). Child and adolescent mental health care in Iran: Current status and future directions. *Archives of Iranian Medicine, 19*(11), 797–804. doi:0161911/AIM.0010

Shooshtari, S., Samadi, S. A., Zarei, K., Naghipur, S., Martin, T., & Lee, M. (2014). Facilitating and impeding factors for knowledge translation in intellectual and developmental disabilities: Results from a consultation workshop in Iran. *Journal of Policy & Practice in Intellectual Disabilities, 11*(3), 210. doi:10.1111/jppi.12084

Siu, A. (2016). Screening for autism spectrum disorder in young children: U.S. Preventive Services Task Force recommendation statement. *JAMA, 315*(7), 691–696. doi:10.1001/jama.2016.0018

Song, Z., Giannotti, T., & Reichow, B. (2013). Resources and services for children with autism spectrum disorders and their families in China. *Infants and Young Children, 26*(3), 204–212. doi:10.1097/IYC.0b013e3182979228

Sousa, A. C. (2011). From refrigerator mothers to warrior-heroes: The cultural identity transformation of mothers raising children with intellectual disabilities. *Symbolic Interaction, 34*(2), 220–243. doi:10.1525/si.2011.34.2.220

Spjut Jansson, B., Miniscalco, C., Westerlund, J., Kantzer, A.-K., Fernell, E., & Gillberg, C. (2016). Children who screen positive for autism at 2.5 years and receive early intervention: A prospective naturalistic 2-year outcome study. *Neuropsychiatric Disease and Treatment, 12,* 2255–2263. doi:10.2147/NDT.S108899

Stein, M. A. (2011). China and disability rights. *Loyola of Los Angeles International and Comparative Law Review, 33*(1), 6–26. Retrieved from http://digitalcommons.lmu.edu/cgi/viewcontent.cgi?article=1658&context=ilr

Steinhausen, H., Jensen, C. M., & Lauritsen, M. B. (2016). A systematic review and meta-analysis of the long-term overall outcome of autism spectrum disorders in adolescence and adulthood. *Acta Psychiatrica Scandinavica, 133*(6), 445–452. doi:10.1111/acps.12559

Tandon, A., Murray, C. J., Lauer, J. A., & Evans, D. B. (2000). *Measuring overall health system performance for 191 countries.* Geneva: World Health Organization.

Thomas, K., Parish, S., Rose, R., & Kilany, M. (2012). Access to care for children with autism in the context of state Medicaid reimbursement. *Maternal and Child Health Journal, 16*(8), 1636–1644. doi:10.1007/s10995-011-0862-1

U.S. Government Printing Office. (2004). *Individuals with Disabilities Education Improvement Act of 2004: Conference report (to accompany H.R. 1350).* (2004). Washington, DC: Author.

United Kingdom National Screening Committee. (2012). *The UK NSC recommendation on Autism screening in children.* Retrieved from https://legacyscreening.phe.org.uk/autism

United Nations Conference on Trade and Development. (2016, September 16). *Classifications.* Retrieved from http://unctadstat.unctad.org/EN/Classifications.html

United Nations Conference on Trade and Development. *Economic groupings and composition* (2016, December 22). *Economic groupings and composition* (Rep.). Retrieved from http://unctadstat.unctad.org/EN/Classifications/DimCountries_EconomicsGroupings_Hierarchy.pdf

Ward, S. L., Sullivan, K. A., & Gilmore, L. (2016). Practitioner perceptions of the assessment and diagnosis of autism in Australia. *Australian Psychologist, 51*(4), 272–279. doi:10.1111/ap.12211

Webb, S. J., Jones, E. H., Kelly, J., & Dawson, G. (2014). The motivation for very early intervention for infants at high risk for autism spectrum disorders. *International Journal of Speech-Language Pathology, 16*(1), 36–42. doi:10.3109/17549507.2013.861018

Wing, L., & Gould, J. (1979). Severe impairments of social interaction and associated abnormalities in children: Epidemiology and classification. *Journal of Autism and Developmental Disorders, 9,* 11–29. doi:10.1007/BF01531288

Wing, L., Yeates, S., Brierly, L., & Gould, J. (1976). The prevalence of early childhood autism: Comparison of administrative and epidemiological studies. *Psychological Medicine, 6,* 89–100. doi:10.1017/S0033291700007522

World Bank. (2014). *Measured approach to ending poverty and boosting shared prosperity: Concepts, data, and the twin goals.* Herndon, VA: World Bank Publications.

World Bank. (2017). *World Bank country and lending groups.* Retrieved from https://datahelpdesk.worldbank.org/knowledgebase/articles/906519

World Health Organization. (2016). *World health statistics 2016: Monitoring health for the SDGs.* Geneva, Switzerland: Author.

Ziats, M. N., & Rennert, O. M. (2016). The evolving diagnostic and genetic landscapes of autism spectrum disorder. *Frontiers in Genetics, 7*(65). doi:10.3389/fgene.2016.00065

Zwaigenbaum, L., Bauman, M. L., Stone, W. L., Yirmiya, N., Estes, A., Hansen, R. L., & Wetherby, A. (2015). Early identification of autism spectrum disorder: Recommendations for practice and research. *Pediatrics, 136*(4 Suppl 1), S10–S40. doi:10.1542/peds.2014-3667C

Index

Printed in the United States
By Bookmasters